When the Words Suddenly Stopped

Finding My Voice Again
After a Massive Stroke

VIVIAN L. KING

Published by Author Academy Elite
P.O. Box 43, Powell, OH. 43035
www.AuthorAcademyElite.com

Identifiers:
LCCN: 2019919214
ISBN: 978-1-64746-056-3 (paperback)
ISBN: 978-1-64746-057-0 (hardback)
ISBN: 978-1-64746-058-7 (ebook)

Available in paperback, hardback, e-book, and audiobook.
All Scripture quotations, unless otherwise indicated, are taken from The Holy Bible, New International Version® NIV® Copyright © 1973 1978 1984 2011 by Biblica, Inc. ^{TM}
Used by permission of Zondervan. All rights reserved worldwide.

Any Internet addresses (websites, blogs, etc.) and telephone numbers printed in this book are offered as a resource. They are not intended in any way to be or imply an endorsement by Author Academy Elite, nor does Author Academy Elite vouch for the content of these sites and numbers for the life of this book.

Interior book design by Jetlaunch.
Cover design by Abdo_96.
Author photo by James Seder Photography.

Dedication

This book is dedicated to my parents, Marilyn and Virgil King, my grandmother, Louise Coleman, and my uncle, David Lester Hawkins, Jr.

Thank you, Mom, for being my constant caretaker and my best friend, even when I did not realize it. Your support means the absolute world to me, and I cannot thank you enough.

Thank you, Daddy—now in heaven—for being my biggest champion and believing and teaching me that I could do anything I put my mind to and that I can do ALL things through Christ.

Thank you, Grandma Louise, also now in heaven, for being a praying grandmother—especially during this ordeal—and always lighting up when I entered your room.

Finally, my Uncle Lester passed away unexpectedly less than six months before I started writing this book, proving that tomorrow is not promised. His best friend says my uncle is beaming in heaven right now.

I am who I am because of all of you, and I love you more than words can express.

Table of Contents

Part I: The Emergency

Part II: The Healing

Part III: The Lessons

Foreword

Miami International Airport was even crazier than usual, but I made it through with time to spare. Being early after battling the crowds brought me a small measure of joy and gave me time to reflect. I'd been overdue for a short vacation, and my friend Vivian convinced me to go somewhere. Anywhere.

As I waited for my connection back home to Chicago, I was eager to tell Viv that once again, she was right. I settled into a much-coveted airport seat and prepared to dial. I grabbed my phone to call Vivian, and at that very moment, it rang.

The caller ID showed "Vivian King."

She wins again. I laughed aloud, fully prepared to give her major points.

I automatically answered.

"Why you calling me? You are always right, Miss King!"

I was actually babbling until the voice on the other end said, "Hosea, it's not Vivian. This is Vivian's friend, June."

Why is she calling me? This can't be good.

"Vivian is in intensive care. She's had a stroke," June said.

At that point, it was like listening to Charlie Brown's teacher. All I heard was, "Wah wa wa wah wa."

I was standing still, but everything around me was in fast motion, swirling. I remember walking toward customer service to change my flight and head from Miami to Milwaukee rather than Chicago, all the while asking the voice on the phone, "How is she? Where is she?"

"It's not good."

My heart dropped.

"I'm on the way," I said.

"Don't come. We have it under control. Her mother will be here soon," said June.

Don't come? I thought but didn't say it because the lady was so adamant.

"I need to be with Vivian!" I did say.

"No. It's best you don't come."

Who the hell was this telling me not to come see about my best friend?

Apparently, she didn't know I'd claimed Viv from the first time I saw her on TV in Alexandria, Louisiana.

"Who is that girl on Channel 5?" I had asked my friend Patrick, whom I was visiting at the time.

I was mesmerized.

"That's my friend Vivian," Patrick said. "I told you about her. We're meeting her for dinner later."

You would have thought I was in Times Square on New Year's Eve! Bells, whistles, balloons, fireworks. I was going to hang out with the most dynamic person I'd seen on the screen in years. Mind you, at this point, I was a news anchor in Los Angeles.

Over dinner, we laughed and shared deep thoughts, then laughed some more. I thought, "She's going to be my friend, whether she likes it or not!"

And she was.

Through the years, we shared secrets, and she called out my rare "fabrications."

We traveled and laughed.

We whispered and laughed.

Advised and laughed.

Talked until the early morning hours, often about nothing, once I think about it.

Vivian was the first person I called with good news, and the first person I called when life dealt me an unforeseen blow.

And I felt honored that she shared with me—a lot.

You see, Vivian puts up a brave and happy front, but she often hid her pain. Except from me.

Lord, we even went to our first nude beach together!

But that's for another book.

And now this lady was telling me that I couldn't come see about my friend?

My Vivian?

Apparently, "the people" thought it was best. And my Vivian could not speak for herself. My talented, gifted, blessed friend could not tell them I needed to be with her, whispering and laughing.

Vivian's words were gone. The laughter went missing.

Now it's all back.

And her old, raggedy friend can't wait to hear her thoughts.

To learn what I missed when her words went away.

Hosea Sanders, Anchor/Reporter
14-Time Emmy Award Recipient
ABC 7 News, Chicago, 2019

A Note from the Author

Dear Reader,

From as early as I can remember, I have wanted to have fun, make a difference, and look good while doing it. Thus, my choices in life have all had that aim.

My friend Hosea always jokingly asks me, "Do you have to be president of *everything?*"

"No," I always answer, "but . . . "

The answer of the day always includes why I decided to pursue the presidency of the latest organization.

This attraction to activity and commitment to service started when I was a child in St. Louis, most likely because my parents exposed their only child to a lot of different experiences. (I have two sisters from my father's first marriage, but they lived with their mother.)

I remember selling Kool-Aid with my next-door neighbor to raise money. I was an active leader with my church youth group. In elementary school, I acted in a theater group that had the goal of developing students in the arts. We performed for each elementary school in the district.

I was also a voracious reader, often reading six books at a time and carrying them all in my backpack—every day. Of course, studies later showed that this was not a good practice for one's back, but how many things did we do back then that would be deemed unsafe or unhealthy today?

I ran track, cross country and played volleyball in middle school. In high school, I was captain of the pom-pom squad and voted "Most Likely to Succeed" by my senior class. I really thought I should be best dressed, but my old boyfriend and another classmate received that honor. I accepted the loss because they *were* always sharp.

My presidential runs began in college. I was president of the Legion of Black Collegians and the Epsilon Psi Chapter of Delta Sigma Theta Sorority. In fact, my sorors, as we call each other in Delta, talked me into trying out for homecoming court. Can you believe I won? Marvin Cobbs and I made history becoming the first African American couple crowned homecoming king and queen of the University of Missouri-Columbia. (My father was always proud of that and would be happy I included this tidbit.) This was quite a rarity at the time because Mizzou, as it's known, was predominantly white, with only two percent of its students being black. Our experience as homecoming couple would need its own book, so I'll move on.

Over the years, I was president of two more Delta Alumnae chapters in Battle Creek, Michigan, and Milwaukee, Wisconsin. I was also president of the Wisconsin Black Media Association, the Black Public Relations Society of Milwaukee, Chair of the Milwaukee Urban League Board, co-chair of its annual

Black and White Ball, and vice-chairs and members of various other civic boards.

When I moved to Milwaukee to work in the news, I really thought I would be out in three years, moving on to the next bigger television market. You see, I had signed a three-year contract at WTMJ-TV, the NBC affiliate in Milwaukee. Two decades and careers later, I am still in Milwaukee. Many of my friends are shocked because they know how much I love big cities and traveling, but two people—independent of each other— said to me when I arrived, "Milwaukee sucks you in. You will probably stay here." Clearly, I thought they were grossly mistaken. It turns out they were right.

Milwaukee has been good to me. I thoroughly enjoyed my television career. Not only did I love what I did—being on the front line of stories and history—but I made lifelong friends. Then, an unexpected and chance career change landed me in a director of public affairs spot for local grocery chain Roundy's Supermarkets. There, I was the primary spokesperson for the company and also promoted the Roundy's Foundation. My work garnered the attention of the largest health care system in Wisconsin at the time, and I became the vice president of community relations at Aurora Health Care.

So, you're probably wondering, *Where is the fun in her life?* I recently read an article by Dan Read entitled "Americans Waste More Than $200 Billion Annually by Failing to Use All Their Vacation Time." That is *not* me. In fact, a co-worker who fits this category gifted me some of *his* vacation days one year.

It was during the early years of my time in Milwaukee that I started traveling a lot, thanks to a childhood friend who was a flight attendant. We first started off with buddy passes for me, but then she named me her companion traveler when single flight attendants were allowed to add a friend or relative who is not a spouse or parent to receive flight benefits. The end result was my getting a passport and using it for trips to Paris, Italy, Amsterdam, Brazil, and Ecuador.

Even after my companion-travel status ended, I continued to travel—to London, on a Mediterranean cruise, back to Italy, on a Caribbean cruise for my fortieth birthday, to the Southern Caribbean a year later, to Las Vegas, Hawaii, and more. As a gift to my parents, I took them to Israel with my church. I have now lived in five states, visited thirty-seven more, and traveled to countries across six continents.

You can probably imagine what my photo Christmas cards have looked like over the years, which is why many of my family and friends have shared that they look forward to my card arriving each holiday season to see the latest country I've visited. One friend's husband calls me "World-Wide."

But now there's Facebook, which allows me to post about my vacations immediately. (Most people think this is unsafe to do, but I take precautions.) My more than 2,000 friends have said they live vicariously through me. They have loved parasailing over Cozumel, touring the Bacardi distillery in San Juan, Puerto Rico, watching me get baptized in the Jordan River, or even zip-lining through the woods of Lake Geneva, Wisconsin. Almost all of them tell me I am photogenic and that I never take a bad picture. I quickly correct them by telling them I never *post* a bad picture. I have to admit I love fashion, and I strive to have my make-up and lipstick on point—having learned tricks of the trade from my years in television. This makes me almost always camera-ready.

My friends probably also used Facebook to try to keep up with the men in my life. I have dated mostly casually over the years and have gone out with good friends to dinner, charity events, or maybe even a Milwaukee Bucks game. One person, pre-Facebook, was in my life off and on for ten years. Then there was Gerald Johnson, who helped my entre into the corporate world, and my friend, Raymond Downs, who I have known since high school and was dating before the words suddenly stopped. My rule has typically been not to go back to a relationship because it ended for a reason, but this seemed different because of our history. Raymond was one of the people I interviewed when I decided to write this book.

At first, I thought there would be a handful of people to interview, but the more I talked to people, the more I learned that I needed to add to the list. I ultimately interviewed twenty-two people. I recorded most of the conversations. As I logged them, I laughed, cried tears of joy, and got chills down my spine. I hope as you read this story, you will feel many, if not all, of the same emotions I felt in recounting this story.

This book details the real-life journey that landed an energetic lover-of-life and a relatively healthy black woman in the hospital for thirty-two days after suffering from a stroke. Part of that hospital stay was in the Neurological Intensive Care Unit, which means I was out of it and not cognizant of much that was happening, especially in the beginning days.

Thus, I relied on the skills and tactics I used every day during my eighteen-year broadcast career. I interviewed the people in my life at the time, particularly those who were at the event where my health issue became apparent, and the family and friends who nursed me back to health. This book will explore what led up to my crisis. Ultimately, though, this story is about faith, family, and friendship, and how all three converged to lead me from trauma to triumph.

With much gratitude!

Vivian L. King

PART 1

The Emergency

CHAPTER ONE

Waking Up on Friday, October 25, 2013

(Written on October 25, 2018)

Five years ago today started out like any other. I woke up, lamented that it was early and that I had to be at a Girl Scouts breakfast by 7:30 a.m., but other than that, I felt fine. The comfort of my bed almost made me text Sadhna to tell her I wasn't going to be able to make it after all, but she had invited me weeks ago. I had to get up and go.

After showering and getting dressed quickly, I rushed out of the house with my purse and makeup bag in hand. I was going to have to do my makeup in the car *again*. Of course, I only do my makeup at stoplights, or in the car at my final destination *if* I haven't finished on the way. In hindsight, my not putting on my makeup was the first unusual thing to happen that day. I arrived at the hotel where the breakfast was taking place, and I walked in, without my makeup.

At the door, they told me my table was in the front, which made sense because Sadhna was a board member. The hostess escorted me to my table. As I entered the ballroom, there were many people I knew who were welcoming me into the room. A "Hi, Vivian" on the right, a "Hey, girl" on the left, complete with a couple of hugs. In my mind, I was returning the greetings as I normally did at these types of events.

Once we arrived at my table, I said hello to Sadhna and sat down in the only empty seat. Sadhna looked at me and said, "Man, I know you were going to get sushi after work yesterday, but you must have tied one on."

I just looked at her.

At that point, a former colleague I worked with at Today's TMJ4 said hello from across the table. Again, I returned the greeting. Someone next to me suggested that I start eating breakfast. I took one bite of sausage, and that's the last thing I remember clearly for nearly ten days.

CHAPTER TWO

The Breakfast

Sadhna Lindvall's office was right next door to mine when we worked together at Aurora Health Care. We were already good friends prior to my being appointed Vice President of Community Relations because we had seen each other in the field for years, as we reported for competing television stations. Sadhna was on my go-to list when I solicited employees to sit at tables as part of the community sponsorships my department oversaw on behalf of our company, so I think inviting me to the Girl Scouts breakfast was her way of returning the favor. I did not see Sadhna right away when I arrived, but I did see my good friend, Genyne Edwards.

Genyne recalls thinking, *Why did I sign up for this breakfast?*

Much like me, Genyne didn't care for early morning events on a Friday. After checking in at the registration table, Genyne saw her table host.

"Who's going to be at the table?" she asked.

She says she was pleased when the hostess mentioned my name as one of the guests and thought, *OK, great. I'm straight.*

Genyne always enjoyed my company.

This breakfast included food stations, so Genyne walked to our table, put down her belongings and headed straight for the coffee station. As she was perusing the breakfast selections, she saw me. Genyne walked up to me, gave me a hug, and said she was happy I had finally arrived.

Genyne told me she looked at me and wondered, *What's going on with Viv?* She noticed I didn't have on any make-up. Genyne kept networking but was alarmed when she saw me again as she got back to the table.

"When I saw you the second time, I looked at your face, and you just weren't yourself. There was no eye contact with me," she said. "You weren't your kind of vivacious, talking-to-everybody self. You were talking to people, but it seemed like you weren't engaging with them a lot." She recalls thinking, *Hmm, that's weird. Something's going on with Viv.*

Sadhna recalled a similar feeling. "When you walked in, you weren't really smiling. You didn't really have a smile on your face," she said. "You didn't look like yourself."

Knowing that I left work the evening before heading to a sushi date with a mutual friend, Sadhna remembered joking with me.

"I said, 'It must've been some night of sushi,' but you didn't laugh—you just kind of looked straight past me. And I thought, *I hope she's not mad.* I was just poking a little fun, I guess."

Nayo Parret, a fellow member of Delta Sigma Theta Sorority, Incorporated, and one of the women I call *soror,* said, "I was actually way on the other side of the room, but I knew you and Genyne were there because when I came in, I saw Genyne and then I saw you, so I said hi."

"I heard people say you didn't seem yourself, and you didn't have your makeup on. What I noticed is that I just thought you were preoccupied, and I went back to my table as the program was about to start."

Genyne Edwards: "I was sitting directly across the table from you. Your back was to the podium. I was facing it. I remember looking over at you again and being like, *Viv is not herself.* I remember you grabbing your drink, picking it up, and right after you picked it up, it fell out of your hand."

Nayo Parret: "I heard the noise from across the room. It seemed like everyone around you heard it at once and stood up as if in unison, to utter a startled 'Oh.' I stood up and thought, *Oh my gosh, that's at Genyne and Vivian's table.* I was concerned something was terribly wrong, and I had the immediate urge to descend on your table to check."

Sadhna Lindvall: "And the next thing I knew, you started to foam at the mouth and started leaning over and collapsed on the floor."

Genyne Edwards: "As soon as I looked and clued in on you, you basically started foaming at the mouth and started grabbing and hitting the table hard. And then the water fell, and then you fell. You got really stiff first, stiff as a board. And you started shaking violently, and then you rolled and fell to the floor."

Sadhna Lindvall: "Everything from that point on seemed a little surreal. I got out my phone and called 9-1-1."

Genyne Edwards: "I was really screaming and out of sorts. And I remember you being on the floor, and you were just convulsing and shaking really hard."

Sadhna Lindvall: "So, you're down on the ground. We were waiting for EMS. It felt like an hour had gone by, but it was probably only like ten to thirteen minutes with all that was happening. It just felt like forever because of all of the conversations and all of the things happening at the same time."

Nayo Parret: "Nobody knew what to do. Somebody was fanning you, and then Genyne asked if I had contact information for your parents, and so I said no, but I can probably find someone who does. I remember my hands shaking as I started going through the contact list of your mobile phone with you passed out as a backdrop."

Genyne Edwards: You had on some boots and some tights and a dress. I remember pulling your dress down."

Deidra Edwards (another friend unrelated to Genyne): "I was at almost the total opposite side of the room, but in the first or second row, and I could tell that something had happened, that something had gone down. When I saw everybody jump up, that's when someone went to the mic and asked if anybody in the room was a doctor or trained in CPR. At first, I didn't go over, but they were panicked. They were frantic. The hotel staff was going back and forth and said they had called an ambulance and that they were on the way.

"What most disturbed me was that the organizers were trying to start the program, but people were like, uh-uh, what is going on. So, I walked over and saw legs and people crowded around you, not fully knowing to whom the legs belonged."

Genyne Edwards: "You were still convulsing, and it was pretty hard and aggressive. And I just remember thinking in my mind, this is taking a really long time for them [the paramedics] to come."

Deidra was still approaching my table.

Deidra Edwards: "I was thinking, *No, this isn't right. If somebody is lying on the floor, you need to give them air. Why is everybody standing around?* Then I realized that the person on the floor was you. And of course, I kneel down, and now I'm over you. I shouted, 'When is somebody coming? What is going on? What happened?'

"Somebody at your table told me you just passed out. They didn't know what happened, that you just lost consciousness. I asked if you had said anything, and I believe somebody said you weren't feeling well. And then you were gone. Unconscious. You seemed to be trying to come out of it a little bit, and then you were just out of it, just out of it. At that point, I went back to my table to get my mobile phone."

Genyne Edwards: "I was relieved when the paramedics finally arrived. You were still on the floor, and I just remember welling up with tears and thinking, *this is horrible,* because you were out of it."

The ballroom was dimly lit, and in the ruckus around my falling, I must have kicked my purse under the table, because no one could find my identification, car keys or anything I had brought with me to the breakfast. The EMS personnel were adamant about having that information before starting treatment.

Across town, Dr. Joan Prince was at her car dealership, getting her car serviced when her iPhone rang.

"I looked down and noticed it was Deidra Edwards calling. I decided to call her back after finishing the conversation I was having with the service attendant. After he walked away, I listened to the voicemail.

"Deidra was hysterical and said, 'I'm at the Girl Scouts breakfast, and Vivian has had some type of episode. The paramedics are here. She fainted, and they believe she's not responsive.' I called her back right away.

"Deidra said, 'Joan, Vivian has had some kind of episode. I understand she was foaming at the mouth, and she's not conscious right now.' And I screamed. I go, 'What? Where are you?' And Deidra said, 'Again, I'm at the Girl Scouts breakfast. The paramedics want to know if anyone knows about her health history.'

"I told Deidra to put one of them on the phone. She put me on speaker. They asked if you had a history of epilepsy or seizures, and I told them you had never said to me that you had a history of epilepsy or seizures. You'd never said that it ran in the family. I told them I had known you ever since you came to Milwaukee, and you had always been healthy. This was all news to me. In fact, you'd never talked to me about a family member having a stroke or dying from a stroke. And the paramedics told me that's what they needed to know.

"I asked them where they were taking you, but the paramedic had already stepped away from the phone. I yelled at Deidra to tell me where they were taking you, and when she asked, the ambulance driver said they wouldn't know until they got in the ambulance. I told Deidra to stay there and to call me as soon as she knew where they were taking you."

The paramedics finally stabilized me and put me on a stretcher. Sadhna began following them as they carried me out of the room.

Sadhna Lindvall: "As I was walking out with the EMS and you, I kept getting stopped by people asking me where they were taking you, and I just kept saying, 'They're taking her to Sinai. They're taking her to the closest hospital.'"

Ironically, Sadhna's and my offices were on the Aurora Sinai Campus.

Genyne was one of the people who asked about which hospital they were taking me.

Genyne Edwards: "I remember telling Nayo, 'Let me grab her purse.' I grabbed your purse, and I remember leaving with Nayo."

Deidra Edwards: "My biggest concern was trying to get as much information as possible before contacting your mother. I did not want her to panic and get upset if this wasn't a major health emergency. However, from the looks of it, people had already determined that it probably was. I remember feeling strange after hearing the paramedics ask if you took birth control pills. I thought, *why would they ask such a thing, especially in a public place?*"

Sadhna Lindvall: "Once the paramedics got outside the hotel, they asked if I wanted to ride in the ambulance with you. Because the hospital was just a few blocks away, I decided to drive on my own. I went to get in my car parked on the street and drove it around to the front hotel driveway behind where the ambulance was parked. For some reason, it didn't move.

"I got out of the car and tried to get into the ambulance, but the paramedics told me I was going to have to wait. You were having another seizure. They said they just needed to stabilize you again, and they would meet me at the hospital. So, I waited. I didn't move until the ambulance moved."

CHAPTER THREE

Deltas on Call

June Perry's day started off as her days typically did after retirement. She was still in her pajamas, in bed, reading the newspaper and watching the morning news. The phone rang, and it was Genyne calling. She was crying.

"June," Genyne exclaimed. "You've got to get here. Something has happened to Vivian. I don't know what happened, but they are taking her to Sinai. Can you go?"

"It was no question if I could go," said June. "It was how long would it take for me to get there. So, I jumped up, put on my clothes and went to the hospital to meet the ambulance."

Joan was still at the car dealership, panicking at this point, which was not like her. She began looking for her salesperson, Chris, who is also her dear friend. When she looked over toward his office, he was not there. So, she took off running, barging into the service bay area after seeing her car hoisted on a service pillar.

"Get my car down. I need it *immediately*. I have an emergency," Joan screamed.

People were looking at Joan like she was insane, but she kept yelling.

"Get my car down. Get it down *now*!" Joan said.

One of the service technicians responded. "Dr. Joan, what's wrong?"

"My girlfriend has had some type of seizure or something," she shouted. "They have called the paramedics. I've got to get to the hospital."

At the same time, her cell phone rang again, and it was Deidra with the news that they were taking me to Sinai. Also, by this time, her salesperson Chris had made it to the service bay.

"Joan, what's wrong?" Chris asked.

Joan, by then, was screaming and crying. "Get my car down, Chris. I gotta GO," she said.

"Get her car down," Chris said.

It took longer than Joan would have liked because they had to put the parts they had taken out back in, which gave Chris time to try to stop Joan from driving to the hospital alone. "Let me drive you," he said. "I don't think you're in the condition to drive."

"I am. I am," Joan responded. "I promise I'll calm down. I'll slow down."

Chris reluctantly agreed to let Joan drive away by herself. She admitted going over the speed limit on her way to Sinai.

"I was in and out of cars, and all I kept thinking was, at that point, I had no idea what was going on," Joan said. "I didn't know if you were conscious. I didn't know if you had died on the spot. I didn't know 'cause they didn't know to tell me."

All Deidra had told Joan was that I was non-responsive. With her background in hematology and having once run a lab, all Joan could think was that health care workers have said someone is non-responsive when they are dead. Nagging in her mind was the question, "What are they not telling me?"

Everybody seemed to be arriving at the hospital in quick succession, either right before or right after the ambulance arrived. And nobody seemed to be observing the parking rules.

Deidra Edwards: "We're all like in there and parking wherever and not paying attention to where we were parking. I think I had parked behind the ambulance."

Sadhna Lindvall: "I had parked legally in the emergency room parking lot. When I got into the emergency waiting room, all of these people were there that I think were called by the people who were asking me where they were taking you. June was there. Genyne was there. We had someone come up and ask if any of us were family or relatives. And they said they could only allow family back there, so June raised her hand and said, 'I'm her sister.' And she went. And I just remember that moment of keeping my mouth quiet."

June actually got to the hospital right before my ambulance. Also, Nayo had joined the contingent, and of course, Deidra.

Genyne Edwards: "June took your purse from me, and she was like down to business. Like, 'I don't have time for you. I'll talk to you later.' I remember her walking up to the desk and walking back through the emergency doors."

So, June was the only one of my friends who was initially allowed to go back to the treatment room with me. She was the only one who witnessed the first series of questions the emergency room doctors were asking me.

June Perry: "They were asking you, 'What day is it? Do you know who the president is?' And you were able to answer when you first came in. Then they started working on you to try to determine what was happening and kept asking you questions. Eventually, you weren't responding.

"And the physician said to me, 'We need to send her to St. Luke's because something is happening, and we're going to try to prevent her from having a stroke.' So that was the whole focus, trying to prevent. But you were slowly losing the ability to respond."

As they prepped me for the trip to St. Luke's, June went back out into the waiting room.

Joan, still on the freeway, contacts another one of our sorority sisters, Jessica Murphy. "Something's going on with Vivian. All I know is that she's passed out." Joan said.

Jessica must have noticed the panic in Joan's voice because she responded, "Calm down. Take a couple of breaths. Keep me posted."

Jessica, in turn, called Nuntiata Buck ("Nuncie," for short), also in my sorority and a reading specialist with the Milwaukee Public Schools (MPS). She was at work when she got several messages.

Nuncie Buck: "Normally, I have my phone on vibrate or in my purse somewhere, but I had taken it out, and it was on my desk. All of a sudden, all I could see was message after message after message of missed calls from random people who I just don't talk to early in the morning like that."

Jessica, Nayo, and Darienne, who was the MPS School Superintendent at the time, all called Nuncie that morning.

"To make a long story short, I had gotten the calls and, on the phone, all they could say was 'Nuncie, where are you?' I said, 'I'm at MPS.' " They told me you had had a seizure and had passed out. It didn't seem real. All I could think was, *Vivian? Vivian ain't sick. Picture of health. Always bubbly, ready to go.* And I said, 'OK, so, where are you?'

"They told me they were at the Girl Scouts breakfast and that they were waiting on the ambulance. I was starting to get frantic because she needed to get to her hospital with the people who would know how to take care of her, so I told them to get her to St. Luke's."

"In the back of my mind, I kept thinking, *she has to have the best care. She has to be taken care of.* And the first thing I asked them is if anyone had talked to your mother and who had done what so far. I grabbed everything I could think of because I knew that passing out wasn't anything good and that I might not be coming back to the office."

I've known Beverly Cooley since I arrived in Milwaukee and began being active with the Milwaukee Alumnae Chapter of Delta Sigma Theta. She was on my committee when I first co-chaired the Delta Memorial Endowment Fund's Annual Literary Luncheon featuring E. Lynn Harris, may he rest in peace. Plus, we were in our chapter's original book club together because of our love of books. We have been close ever since, and I usually just call her Bev. She was teaching a Weight Watcher's class when she got a call from Nayo Parret.

Beverly said that Nayo asked, "Do you happen to have Vivian's mother's phone number?"

"Why do you need Vivian's mom's phone number?" Beverly asked very deliberately, feeling that it was unusual for Nayo to ask.

That's when Nayo explained that she was at this breakfast with me, that I looked like I had a seizure, and they had brought me to Sinai.

"I knew that as soon as I wrapped up my class, I was headed to the hospital to find out what was going on," Beverly said.

Beverly did not have my mother's phone number, either.

Joan finally reached Highland Avenue from the freeway and pulled off to get to Sinai.

"I come pulling into the ER parking lot. I jump out of the car. I run in, and in the room sitting there are June, Sadhna, and Nayo," said Joan. "I just stand there, and June looks at me and says, 'We don't know yet. They just got her in here. They're in the back.' "

Sadhna was crying.

"Just tell me if she's alive or not," Joan said. "They all replied, 'yes.' "

"But we need to reach her parents," said June.

Joan nodded and told them that she had the phone number. You can't have cell phones in the emergency room, so Joan headed to the area between the emergency room and the parking lot. Before she walked out, she turned to them.

"You guys come and get me when we can go in to see her," Joan said.

"They told me only one person could go back," June replied.

"You go, June," Joan said. "But we're all sisters, so put us down as sisters."

"Got it," said June.

CHAPTER FOUR

A Mother's Worst Nightmare

As a veteran television journalist, I have used the phrase, and so have many of my colleagues—"a mother's worst nightmare." It is a cliché, no doubt, but October 25, 2013, was definitely *my* mother's worst nightmare.

My mom calmly relayed the story five years later. "A policeman came to the door, and Virgil [my father] went to the door because I was in the bathroom. When I got out, he told me a policeman had come to the door and said that a lady named Joan tried to reach us and hadn't been able to and called the police."

Joan had just left the emergency room at Sinai to call my parents. She grabbed her phone and was shaking so much that she couldn't find the number. She then realized that she did not have the home number. Instead, she had my parents' address, which she had gotten from a previous Christmas card. That's when she decided to call the St. Louis police.

"Hi, my name is Joan Prince. This really is not a crank call. I have a friend who is from there. Her parents live there. I'm calling from Milwaukee, Wisconsin. She's had some kind of seizure or something. She's non-responsive, and I don't have the phone number for her parents, but I have an address."

Joan was still nervous. Her voice was shaking, but she said the woman on the line was so kind.

'It's OK. Calm down. Give me the address," the dispatcher said.

Joan provided the address.

"We don't have that address," said the dispatcher.

Joan began feeling the panic starting to rise in her body again.

"Yes, you do have the address," she shouted. "Look it up *again!*"

Joan didn't remember if she had said place or street, but she remembered there was a slight discrepancy in the address she had given to the operator, but the operator figured it out.

"That's actually not in St. Louis. It's in University City," replied the dispatcher. "I have to transfer you over to them. Now, if for *any* reason we get cut off, I'm going to give you my name and a direct number."

"I don't have a pen," said Joan.

"That's OK," the operator said. "I'm going to call you back in five minutes to make sure you're connected."

"They were wonderful," said Joan. "So, they transferred me over, and I remember when the transfer call was made, she said, 'Hello, this is the St. Louis Police Department 9-1-1 Dispatch. I have a woman on the line, Joan Prince. She is calling about Vivian King. We're going to need you to make a home visit to inform her parents that their daughter is ill.

This person is calling from Milwaukee, Wisconsin. She does not have their phone number.'

"So, she was able to make the transfer and the call," Joan said. "Then the people in University City were so kind, and they said, 'We're going to contact an officer who's in the field and have him go to the house, but we're going to keep you on the line so you'll be able to hear him.'"

At that time, Joan recalled being nervous about how the officer would approach the situation. "But ma'am, when you talk to the officer, I don't want him to say anything bad," Joan said. "The dispatcher responded, 'no, no, no. We handle this all the time.'"

Once contact was made with an officer in the field, Joan heard him walk up to my childhood home. There was a pause while the officer rang the doorbell. Then she heard the door open and my father's voice.

"Are you Virgil King?" the officer said.

"Yes, I am," my father replied.

"I have a Joan Prince from Milwaukee on the phone," the officer said. "She is trying to reach you, and it's in regard to your daughter, Vivian."

Mom later remembered that as Dad relayed the story back to her a few moments after that, he said his heart just dropped at the initial news. That is probably why Joan was so concerned about the officer's initial approach.

"She's had some sort of health attack," the officer said. "But she's alive."

Then he suddenly remembered that he had Joan on the phone.

"Oh, and I have her [Joan] here," he said. "She can hear you, and can you give her your phone number?"

Back in the corridor of the emergency room in Milwaukee, Joan quickly motioned to either Nayo or Sadhna that she needed a pen. She had left her purse inside the waiting room.

"They brought it to me, and that's how I got the info," she said.

My father repeated our phone number and then asked for Joan's number. That's how the first call ended.

Dad was sitting on the bed when my mother came out of the bathroom and asked who was at the door. He told Mom that the policeman came over to tell them that Joan wanted them to call her because I was in the hospital.

"So, we called her," said Mom. "She said that you were in the hospital, that you had been at a breakfast event and had passed out, that some of your friends had called the ambulance, and they took you to Aurora."

"She must have told me that you had a stroke," Mom continued. "She said you weren't talking, but you were awake. She asked if I was coming up. I told her I would call when I got a flight."

"After I got off the phone, I told your Daddy," Mom said.

"Well, I guess we have to get you out of here tomorrow," he said.

"No, *today*," Mom said.

There was not a direct flight from St. Louis to Milwaukee until that evening. This turned out to be a blessing in disguise because my mother was the caregiver for my 98-year-old grandmother, Louise, and my father, who had the beginning signs of dementia as a result of being diagnosed with Parkinsonism, a condition with similar symptoms to Parkinson's disease. The delay gave her time to prepare some meals to keep in the freezer and to call some of her friends who could check on my father and grandmother while my mother made the trip to Milwaukee.

"I started cooking so I could leave food for your grandmother and Daddy," said Mom. "After I started cooking and got several meals together, I put my things in a bag and got cleaned up. I called [Joan] back, and she told me that June would pick me up from the airport."

Joan was so relieved to have reached my parents. She could tell from hearing my father's voice that he was upset. She says my mother appeared calmer when she was able to speak with her. In hindsight, she just remembers thanking God for the contact.

After the call, Joan went back into the emergency room waiting area and realized June had gone back into the treatment room with me. She talked with Sadhna and Genyne for a bit, at which point June re-emerged.

"This is not a Trauma One," said June. "They need to take her to St. Luke's."

Joan reported that she had reached my mother and that my mother would call back as soon as she was able to book a flight. Until the next stop, which was the Neurological Intensive Care Unit (NICU) at Aurora St. Luke's Medical Center, the contingent at Aurora Sinai Medical Center just waited.

June took this downtime to step away and call my friend, Raymond Downs. Raymond went to University City High School with me. We dated back then (and later off and on) and had reconnected that year leading up to our high school reunion. We had a whirlwind year. I had been to California, where he lived at the time, twice. He had been to Milwaukee once. We had met in St. Louis for our reunion, spending time with classmates and family, and we had just celebrated our birthdays together in New York. (We are both Libras.)

When Raymond visited me in Milwaukee that summer, we had dinner at June's place. I believe this is why June felt compelled to call him, even though Deidra and Nuncie strongly expressed that he was not my husband and did not need to know anything at this point.

"I was at home," Raymond said. "I knew something was up with you. I thought there was a surprise. I wasn't thinking something negative. I didn't think what I was gonna hear."

Raymond said June was very calm when she shared limited information about my emergency. "So, at first, I didn't think it was that serious," he said.

It was not until much later that Raymond realized just how serious my situation was.

CHAPTER FIVE

A Serious Situation

Finally, it was time to head to St. Luke's. I had actually only been at Aurora Sinai for about an hour. Nobody was going back to the Girl Scouts breakfast. Since June had told them earlier that she was my sister, she was able to ride in the ambulance with me. Joan followed the ambulance to St. Luke's. The others made their way to their cars to meet me there. Nayo had to walk back through the hospital to get to where her car was parked.

"I remember somehow I was walking through the hallway, and I saw two nurses pushing you," Nayo recalls, "and I looked at you, and you had no recollection of anything. I said, 'hey' while you were passing me, and it was like you looked right through me and didn't see me. I just broke down and started crying. I really thought you were gone.

"I called Priscilla, another one of our sorority sisters. She was trying to comfort me, and I said, 'Priscilla, this is really bad.' I explained what happened, and Priscilla said, 'I wonder if it was a stroke.' "

On a side note, I used to joke with Priscilla all of the time that she got her M.D. from Google.

"I told Priscilla I didn't think so because I didn't recognize any of the telltale signs of someone experiencing a stroke: drooping of the face, weakness in one arm, or difficulty speaking."

Riding in the ambulance, June said she was able to establish a rapport with the paramedics.

"So, when we got to St. Luke's, they kept talking to you, and the guy said, 'We can do things to prevent her from having a stroke. That's what we're focused on.' So, when people would ask me, I would say, 'There's something going on, but we're not sure of what it is. But they are working hard to try to prevent a stroke.' "

It ultimately ended up being a stroke. A blood clot developed on the left side of my brain over the part that manages speech. It bled out, killing all the brain cells in that area. As a result, I could not speak.

June continues. "Eventually, you were nonverbal, and you were not responding to questions, so there was a difference between what was happening at Sinai when you first came in and what was happening at St. Luke's. At that point, it was touch and go because you were totally non-responsive."

Joan is the one who thought to call the pastor of my church. I attend Christ the King Missionary Baptist Church, where John Wesley McVicker, Sr. is the pastor and a good friend. He and his wife, Marilynn—in our denomination's tradition, we call her the First Lady of the church—visited me together. (Ironically, she has the same name as my mother, but she spells her name with a second "n.")

Pastor McVicker: "We identified ourselves, and they allowed us to come into your room. When we saw you, your features were the same. There was no contortion of your face or that you couldn't move or anything like that."

Marilynn McVicker: "I was shocked when I went in, and I had to be strong. You looked weak, and you weren't the Vivian that I'm accustomed to seeing. You were lying there, limp. You needed to have serious care, and that alone blew my mind."

Pastor McVicker: "You had a look on your face like you weren't present. You were physically there. You were awake, but the stare, the look on your face was like you weren't there, like you were mentally detached from what was going on. You were not trying to communicate at all."

Marilynn McVicker: "When I saw you in the bed, and you couldn't speak, that right there made me think, *wait a minute, this is a girl that's always talking, and that's her profession, communicating.* I couldn't get over the fact that that was not available to you and how the brain works. You weren't the Vivian that I'm accustomed to seeing, somebody who was communicating and just full of life."

So, Pastor asked everyone in the room to hold hands, and he prayed. Nobody can remember the actual prayer these many years later, but he most certainly asked God to heal me and restore me to the Vivian I once was.

Once Jessica learned I was at St. Luke's, she left work and went to pick up Beverly.

"As we were entering the building, June was coming out," said Jessica. "She told us where you were and where to find you."

As they were making their way downstairs to the Neurological ICU, they ran into Pastor McVicker.

Jessica told me, "Beverly said, 'We ain't got to worry about nothing.' Pastor McVicker prayed. It's a done deal. Our girl is gonna be OK.' "

Jessica and Beverly checked in with the nurse as soon as they got to the NICU, which is on the lower level of St. Luke's. The nurse told them to sit in the waiting room. By then, they were letting a few people in to see me one at a time because of the other people who were already there with me.

"They asked who we were," said Jessica. "We both immediately said we're her sisters. They did not question it, and they took us to the room."

Beverly remembered going in by herself first. "You did not look like yourself. You looked sick. You looked really sick. All of this equipment and tubes were around you. Your skin didn't look right. Before I saw you, I wasn't really scared. I was on adrenaline. When I saw you, that is when I got scared."

Jessica had a similar experience the first time she laid eyes on me in the hospital. "It took our breath away to see you in the condition you were in. The doctor came in, and since he thought we were your sisters, he told us in detail what was going on. He said that your brain was hemorrhaging and that they needed to stop the bleeding. He told us he needed us to help ask you questions, which would aid them in determining what was going on with your brain.

"So, at that point, we asked you some questions. You just kind of smiled and nodded your head yes or no. We could tell it wasn't really clicking with you. You *did* know your name, and you knew that you stayed on East Locust, but that's about all you said."

Jessica recalled my getting frustrated at some point during this exercise. "We just stopped and took a break. We had to leave the room because it was kind of emotional for us."

At some point during the morning, one of June's calls was to Kimberly Montgomery. Kim and I met at a sorority meeting when I first arrived in Milwaukee in an ironic way. Her Aunt Rubye worked with my mother at the time and had told me to look up her niece, also a member of Delta Sigma Theta, when I moved to town. I had yet to do that, but this chance meeting saved me the trouble.

We were at the meeting those many years ago and ended up sitting next to each other when I was introduced. When she found out that I was from St. Louis, she mentioned that she had an aunt who lived there. I looked in her face and instantly said, "Rubye Davis is your aunt." She looked *just like* Rubye. We have been good friends ever since.

Kim got the call from June and immediately got in her car to come see me. By the time she arrived, I was at St. Luke's. "You were in ICU. They were changing shifts, so I was able to come in and see you. I asked what room you were in, and I was led straight to your room. When I received the call from June, they weren't quite sure what actually triggered your incident. I did not know it was a stroke."

On the way, Kim had taken the time to call her sister and stop and buy a get-well card. When she arrived at the hospital, she had a couple of cards with her, one from her and one from her sister. I am close to her entire family.

"You were sitting in the room, and as I walked in and said 'hello,' you smiled at me with a look of affirmation as though you knew who I was."

As she told me this story, my mind conjured up the memory. The moment came back to me with such clarity.

Kim said, "You were just like now, shaking your head and smiling. I told you that I brought you a couple of cards, and you smiled."

Kim handed me the cards, and I first just held them in my hands. I did not open them. I did not act as though I was going to read them. That is when my symptoms began to ring familiar with Kim.

"Having witnessed my father having a stroke previously and myself experiencing what they call TIA (a transient ischemic attack, often called a mini-stroke because it has similar symptoms as a stroke, yet only lasts a few minutes and causes no permanent damage), I knew the symptoms you were exhibiting were similar to symptoms of a stroke," said Kim. "I recognized then that you didn't know what to do with the cards."

Kim continued. "So, I asked you, 'Well, Vivian, do you want me to open the cards for you?' And you smiled at me again."

"At least, I was friendly," I interjected, and we both laughed.

"You were friendly," Kim said, with levity in her tone. "So, I knew then how to communicate with you, because of what I had witnessed in the past."

Kim said I smiled at her, and she proceeded to open the cards. As she opened the first one, out fell a magnet she had bought. It was a picture of Michelle Obama. I smiled at the magnet when I saw it, but that's all I did, according to Kim.

"Do you want me to read the cards?" Kim asked.

I smiled at her, and so Kim began reading.

"Michelle Obama says get better," Kim read.

Kim then read the card from her sister, Angie Montgomery. Kim sat there for a while with me, talking the entire time. She said I constantly smiled at her, but I did not speak one word. She shared that she feels that's how we know actions speak louder than words. She knew how to communicate with me even though I was not speaking.

After that visit, Kim learned that I indeed had suffered a stroke. Kim felt she is one of the fortunate ones who got to see me, and she believes God allowed it because of her previous experience with strokes. Once she left, what my friends now affectionately call "the shutdown" was about to take place.

Back in the waiting room, Jessica and Beverly began discussing my situation. Jessica describes herself as bossy. We just accept her for who she is.

"This is really serious. Vivian is loved by everybody, but we gotta get a team together," Jessica told Beverly. "I can't have people in and out. I don't want her exposed to everybody in the condition that she's in. So, we will come up with the names of people who I can trust. We'll come up with a shift, and we will just shut it down and not allow people to come in."

Jessica was responding to something else the doctor had said. He had told them I was in serious condition. He wanted to limit the contact I had until my medical team could get a handle on what exactly was going on inside my brain. Echoing in Jessica's mind were the words, *we've gotta get her brain to stop hemorrhaging.*

Beverly had another reason for wanting to limit contact in those early hours. "We started limiting people because we knew you would not want people to see you like this."

It was at about this time that Nuncie arrived at St. Luke's. With limits on contact, my doctors' orders, and the wishes of my friends, Nuncie launched into full protection mode as soon as she hit the hospital doors.

"We went to the triage nurses, all the nurses who were there, and explained we're her sisters." Nuncie spoke on behalf of all my sorority sisters, and the core team she and my "sisters" were beginning to assemble, to advocate for me during this health scare. She went on to tell them that I had never been sick like this to their knowledge. She also remembered capturing some notes so that they could relay any pertinent information to my mother upon her arrival.

Then she and Jessica started working on a schedule. They developed an entire Excel spreadsheet. They looked at who they could trust and who was available to take care of everything they could think of, like transportation for my mother once she arrived at the airport, transportation for Mom to and from the hospital each day, food when she wasn't at the hospital, and whether she would sleep at my condominium or someone else's home. It was fall and starting to get cold in Milwaukee. Plus, they did not want my mother to have to worry about anything other than making sure I was receiving the care I needed.

The people included on the schedule were my mother, of course, and all my "sisters." My sisters included June, Joan, Jessica, Beverly, Nuncie and Grant, another sorority sister who shared season tickets to the Milwaukee Bucks basketball team with Beverly and me. My friend, Tracey Golden, is not my sorority sister, but we consider ourselves sisters in Christ, having first met at Christ the King Baptist Church. We are close. She was on the list. Of course, my pastor and his wife stayed on the list. This left a lot of people out of the loop, which created some hurt feelings I had to deal with after I recovered, but the immediate goal was to limit the distractions so my brain could begin to heal.

"The doctors were great," said Joan. "They would tell us the swelling is down, and the idea was just to get the swelling down because the swelling was on your speech center."

My doctors did not believe my speech center was totally damaged. They just wanted to get the swelling of my brain down so they could evaluate and start the healing process. In the meantime, a neurosurgeon was on standby - just in case the swelling did not subside.

Nayo had left the hospital early on but came back after Grant got off work. "Grant and I got your keys. I had your coat and purse. Grant drove me to pick up your car from the hotel, and then I drove your car to your house. That night we kinda knew it was going to be a long recovery."

My "sisters" were in and out all day over several hours, while other people were calling them on their cell phones and trying to get through to me by calling the hospital. They were asking the obvious questions based on what they had heard through the grapevine, "Well, did she have a stroke?" and "What's going on?"

Jessica would respond, "We're not saying 'stroke.' We don't know what the prognosis is yet." She started getting offended at the questions because she felt that people were prying, and she did not want to spread gossip or misinformation. "I started saying, 'It's very serious' and telling people that when your mom arrived, we would let her decide how she wanted to disseminate information. We were just there until your mom came and could make major decisions for you."

Jessica repeated that mantra to our other sorority sisters and friends. "Then, Beverly went home. Joan called me and said June was picking your mom up at 9 p.m., and she would get there by 10 p.m. I said, 'Well, I can't leave Mother King by herself. I guess I'm gonna spend the night.' "

Jessica settled in for the long haul.

My mother arrived in town on schedule, at about 9 p.m. on Friday. June was assigned to pick her up, and she was right on time.

"Once in Milwaukee, June pulled up, and we went straight to the hospital," Mom said. "At the hospital, I walked over to you, and your eyes were open, and I kissed you. I didn't say anything. You seemed to recognize me. You looked OK. You didn't look like you had had a stroke. You really didn't look bad at all."

Jessica greeted my mother and said, "I'm spending the night with you."

Mom said, "OK."

What happened next was a long, eventful night after what had been a day full of unexpected surprises.

CHAPTER SIX

LBVS (Laughing but Very Serious)

There is typically humor in everything in life. We found that to be true, even with my being in a hospital bed in the Neurological Intensive Care Unit at St. Luke's and especially after my mother arrived that first night.

Jessica remembered how uncomfortable it was the first night after she agreed to stay in the room with my mother. She was in one chair and my mother was in another, and they were pulling up other chairs to try to make it more like a bed. Nothing was working, particularly because my nurses were in the room around the clock, but this routine had started earlier in the day.

"When we first got to the hospital, Beverly and I, you were awake, and then you started moving around," Jessica said. "Beverly was like, 'Does she want something?' And I said, 'I don't know.' "

Nuncie was there, as well. So, the three of them got closer to the bed, looked in, and noticed that I had wet the bed.

"Our sister's wet the bed," they said after buzzing the nurse. "You need to change the sheets."

The nurse went to retrieve clean sheets and came back to change them.

"Are you guys giving her a lot of fluids?" Jessica asked.

They responded that they were giving me fluids through an IV.

"If that's the case, how many times are you going to come in with a bedpan?" Jessica asked. "'Cause she's not getting out the bed, right?"

"Well, when she's gotta go, we'll check on her," the nurse responded.

Jessica insisted that since I could not really speak at this time that I could not tell them when I had to go to the bathroom. The nurse seemed to brush this off yet finished changing the sheets and left. About an hour later, I started moving around again.

"We were just talking, wasting time," said Jessica. "We looked up, and you had taken the cover *off* of you, turned around, and your bare butt was up in the air."

"What the heck is going on?" Beverly asked in horror.

"I think she's got to go to the bathroom, but she can't get up," Jessica said. "So, we ran to the bed, and we covered you up. And before we could walk away, you took the cover back off and had turned around."

This time, Nuncie tried to cover me up with the sheets.

"Why is her butt always facing the door?" Beverly cried out, "We can't have her mooning people."

"No, we can't," Nuncie and Jessica agreed.

They pressed the call button and practically demanded that the nurse come back in quickly because they thought I was motioning that I needed to use the bathroom. The nurse came in, helped me use the bedpan, and then began to leave.

"Well, should you leave the bedpan here?" Jessica asked. "If you show us how to put her on it, we can help."

"No, no, no. She just got here," the nurse said. "We don't want her on the bedpan."

They were not sure why my just getting there was a factor.

"A little over an hour later, you had wet the bed again and was throwing the cover off," said Jessica. "And Beverly said, 'up, there she goes again, taking the cover off her.' I said, 'Oh my God, we can't have her cheeks up in the *air*. That's why we can't have people in here.' "

"Oh, God. If Vivian doesn't stop it," Beverly said, shaking her head. "I don't want to see her little butt in the air."

"I know but what are we supposed to do?" said Jessica as she, Beverly and Nuncie pondered how to keep me from putting on a show for any and everyone who happened to pass my room when it was time for me to "go."

Fast forward to about 10 p.m. that Friday. Beverly and Nuncie had gone home, and Jessica was in my hospital room alone, waiting for my mother to arrive. Once she did, Jessica informed her that she was spending the night so my mother would not have to be alone with me. Jessica also shared with Mom my routine of communicating that I had to go to the bathroom. After I wet the bed about three times because the nurses didn't get there in time, due to their helping other patients, my mother got a little tired of the scenario.

"How many times has she wet the bed?" Mom asked.

"Several," Jessica answered. "And she's been doing some other things, too."

"Like what?" Mom asked.

"Never mind, Mom. You don't want to know," Jessica said, thinking back to my mooning episodes.

By the time a nurse had come in a couple of times to change my sheets, my mother and Jessica had talked one of them into leaving a bedpan. Additionally, they had developed a system of maneuvering me onto the bedpan to use the bathroom.

"We figured it out because at that point, you were not shy about pulling up your hospital robe, being the full monty," said Jessica.

"Oh, Vivian, don't you have any modesty?" my mother said.

"Mom, you don't even want to know the half of it," Jessica said.

After doing this almost every half hour, my thin hospital robe had accidentally gotten a little wet.

"This is not working," Jessica said.

They buzzed the nurse again.

"She didn't wet the bed, but her robe is wet," they said.

The nurse came in again. My mother and Jessica had decided that this was getting to be a bit too much. I was up every half hour. They were up every half hour. I couldn't sleep. They couldn't sleep.

"I don't know why they don't have a catheter for her," Jessica said.

If you've ever been to a hospital to visit a friend or loved one, you may know that a catheter is a flexible hollow tube used to drain fluids from the body. In most cases, it is used to drain urine from the bladder. When the nurse came in, they finally asked her about it.

"Can you guys put her on a catheter?" they asked.

"Well, we asked her earlier if she wanted one, and she told us, no," the nurse responded.

Mom's and Jessica's eyes both got wide, and they responded loudly and in unison.

"She doesn't know what she's saying! You guys better order her a catheter."

"Well, we've got to call the doctor and find out if it's OK," the nurse said.

"Yeah, you do that," Jessica said sarcastically. "She's emptied three bags of fluid. It's coming right through her. She needs a catheter because she's not resting."

"And neither are *we*," Mom said.

Once they put the catheter on me, I was able to sleep. Mom and Jessica were able to sleep. It was a much happier setting. They didn't have to worry about my throwing the covers off me for the rest of the night, or for the rest of my hospital stay for that matter.

When Beverly came back to the hospital the next day, Jessica made the proud announcement.

"Beverly, you don't have to worry about Vivian throwing the cover off of her anymore," Jessica said. "They've gotten her a catheter."

"Thank the Lord," Beverly said. " 'Cause I didn't want to see her butt up in the air all day."

Then Beverly looked at me in my non-responsive state. "Ooh, Vivian, just wait 'til you get out," said Beverly. " 'Cause we're gonna have some stories to tell *you*."

The room erupted in laughter.

My mother stayed with me for the first full week before taking a short trip back to St. Louis to check on my father and grandmother. She told me that even though I could not speak, I never really lost my personality. On one of those days, she was there, feeding me, and I wanted to eat my dessert before the main course.

"Let's wait until you eat the rest of your dinner," Mom said.

I kept resisting.

"No, let's finish your dinner," she repeated.

That's when I, apparently, rolled my eyes at her.

"I know you're not rolling your eyes at me," Mom said.

I made a sound that resembled a sheepish laugh. She said it was as if I knew I was busted. I ate a little more, and then Mom let me have my dessert.

Now, about all my "sisters." One of the things about being single and living in a town away from your family is that your emergency contact does not live with you. Additionally, that person typically does not even live in the same city. Thus, the need for "sisters."

From the beginning of my medical emergency, the hospital staff told the people who began following me from the Girl Scouts breakfast to the emergency room that only immediate family could be in the room with me. That is when my additional sisters were born.

"We told the ICU nurse, we gave her the names of your 'sisters,' " said Joan. "We said, 'Well, our father was very active.' "

"Then she just started looking like, *none of y'all look alike,*" said Nuncie. "She looked over at Joan, looked at me, looked at Jessica, looked at Beverly. It was hilarious. We didn't say a word the first day."

We all laughed as they relayed this story to me.

"And thank goodness it was a sister [African American woman] at the desk writing names," said Joan. "I thought to myself, *they know none of us look alike, but it's OK.* To be culturally sensitive, you can't ask me how I'm related."

Joan felt because this ICU nurse was African American, she might understand our culture and dilemma. Even after those first few days, Nuncie would be in and out of my room during the daytime if she had to visit a school on the south side during the course of her job at MPS. Then the rest of my core team took turns sitting with me during the evening.

Jessica said, "We wanted to make sure you were covered every day, which prompted more nurses to ask, 'How many sisters do you guys have?' I told them, 'We don't look like we're sisters, but she has quite a few sisters. There are at least six of us.' "

The nurses finally stopped questioning my care team, and they did not volunteer any further information. We laughed, thinking back to our image of my nurses who must have thought, "Papa was a rolling stone, wherever he laid his hat was his home," so aptly sung by the Temptations back in 1972, about a man with many children outside his marriage.

Many of my "sisters" got a kick out of some of the answers I gave when my doctors were asking me repeated questions, trying to assess how my brain was functioning.

Beverly Cooley: "At the beginning, when the doctors were asking you questions, you were off on dates, but when they asked you who the president was, you said, 'Barack Obama.' We all laughed because we said, 'Well, she didn't forget that.' "

June Perry: "Even in the emergency room, doctors asked you those same questions: name, address, and current date. An interesting moment was when you answered 'yes' to when the emergency room doctors asked if you could be pregnant. We got a little chuckle out of that, but the situation was still too serious."

Beverly Cooley: "It wasn't like the doctors could tell us much," said Bev. "I think they were trying to manage expectations. We were still in shock that you even had a stroke."

Nuncie Buck: "The second day, [the ICU nurse] came in and said they needed to run diagnostics. Brain function was going all the way back to none. 'She's gonna have to go through therapy, basically having to recondition her mind, her brain, her body to learn things almost as if she was just coming out of a womb' was not something anybody wanted to hear at that time, but we knew we had to stay strong."

Beverly Cooley: "The doctors were telling us, 'You may have to get used to a new normal for Vivian.' None of us could ever see you being any way other than who you were before the stroke."

Nuncie Buck: "And Vivian, the first time you looked up at me in the bed, you just had this stare like, *hmmm, you have a pleasant face, but who are you?* You didn't get scared of us, thank God. You didn't resist, but you just had that look like, *OK, this is another face.*"

Nuncie's education background kicked in at that point, and she asked the nurse to get her a whiteboard and a marker. The nurse agreed. Beverly and Jessica looked on, wondering what Nuncie was about to do.

"We just wanted to see if you remembered anything or could do anything." I wrote on there, 'What's your name?' You took the pen as if you were going to do some regular journaling, and then you just kinda started scribbling. You did some scribbles, but you did not write anything."

The nurse pointed out that my inability to communicate was what concerned them. However, being the encouraging educator who sees good in all her students, Nuncie felt in her mind, *at least she's alert and ready to receive us.*

"Clearly, I can't leave Milwaukee," said my friend and soror, Michelle Greene, as we finally connected via phone for her to provide input for this book.

"You had a stroke. Now Beverly has cancer," Michelle said. "If you two didn't want me to leave, you could've just *told* me."

We broke out into laughter, our normal course, when it comes to our conversations. Michelle is what I call a corporate jet setter. She has lived and traveled all over the world with her growing career in information technology. Furthermore, she is a hoot and has always made me laugh about something.

Michelle and I met years ago during her first stint in Milwaukee. Since then, career opportunities have sent her to Holland, Michigan, back to Milwaukee, and to Detroit (at the time of writing this book), yet she has kept a place in Milwaukee for a variety of reasons. Thus, Michelle's initial joke refers to the two separate times she left Milwaukee. (*Note: Beverly is a cancer survivor, thank God.*)

Michelle was on a flight back to Holland from a business trip when Beverly texted her about my situation, and they actually spoke before her flight took off. Michelle describes her first reaction.

"Of course, very nervous. Then I was grateful that it happened where it did," Michelle said. "I was thinking that if you were home by yourself, how long would it have been before people figured out you had not gone someplace? You're just like me in that respect."

Michelle's first inclination was to figure out how quickly she could get back to Milwaukee. She worked for Johnson Controls, headquartered in Milwaukee, so she could easily be at work and visit the hospital for a few hours. Michelle always traveled with her laptop, so it was easy for her to let her boss know what had happened so she could visit me. She made it to St. Luke's within my first week there, while I was still in ICU.

"I was giving you a hard time because your mom had to come up there," Michelle said.

"I can't believe Vivian did not have her house in order," Michelle said to my mother.

I hated to clean my room as a child. There was always something better to do. This, unfortunately, has seeped into my adult life.

Then Michelle turned to look at me.

"I'm gonna get you when you get better," Michelle said.

Everybody in the room laughed, including the nurses.

"Part of that was trying not to be so heavy the whole time because it was tough. It was overwhelming," Michelle said.

Michelle would end up visiting me in the hospital three or four times. One time, she remembered walking with me around the nurses' station in the ICU, which was situated in the center of the area. Walking the floor meant you walked in a square, as if it were a square track. Private patient areas partitioned off by curtains lined the perimeter.

Another time she visited, she brought our friend, Karla, another soror who worked with Michelle at Johnson Controls. My not being able to communicate was the most shocking aspect of this experience for Michelle, but like all my other supporters, she was not giving up on my recovery.

"Knowing your energy and spirit," said Michelle. "I was not going to sit there and claim that you weren't going to come back from this."

CHAPTER SEVEN

The TV Sisterhood

Remember the book (and later the movie) *Divine Secrets of the Ya-Ya Sisterhood?* The novel came out in 1996, but we saw it at the movies in 2002, and that's when Susan, Katrina, Kim, and I decided to call ourselves the TV Sisterhood. Not because our lives necessarily resembled the characters in the book and movie, but because the story is about friendship—how it changes over time yet can still remain strong.

We all met when we worked at WTMJ-TV together. They arrived in 1994. I came along a year later. Susan Kim was a morning anchor by this time. Katrina Cravy is our "California Girl" who left us for Portland but came back and worked for our competitor before leaving television, writing a book, and starting a business. Kim Buchanan, the producer, was our organizer of all things. She now executive produces a talk show at the station and still pays attention to all details. Then there I was: a former education reporter–turned anchor–turned grocery chain spokesperson–turned community relations vice president.

Between job changes, marriages, and kids, we may not talk every day, but we are still good friends and are there for each other. That's why my medical incident rocked them to their core. Like when the characters of the Ya-Ya Sisterhood rushed in and revealed their secrets to help salvage the relationship between their "sister" Viviane and her daughter, my TV Sisterhood wanted to rush in and save me.

As we sat laughing and catching up more than five years after my stroke, we feasted on our favorite collective dinner, sushi. After family updates, we finally got down to discussing my stroke and who heard the news first.

Katrina Cravy: "I got the information from Kim."

Kim Buchanan: "I got it from you." She pointed to Susan.

Susan Kim: "I saw it on Facebook. I freaked out and then texted Kim."

Kim Buchanan: "And then I called you [Susan] because I was outside on the phone. And you were like, 'apparently, nobody's heard from her.' "

Because my episode happened on a Friday, we were trying to figure out when, exactly, they tried to come to see me. I say *try* because the decision had already been made to curtail my visitors to help my brain heal. Regardless, after Susan talked with Kim, she called Aurora Sinai, where they told her they could not give out any patient information. She then called my cell phone, and whoever was with me answered and said I was now at St. Luke's.

Susan Kim: "I called you at St. Luke's on the telephone, and you answered. And I remember texting Kim, 'She sounds great,' though you did not sound totally like yourself. Did it seem like you were 100% aware of what our conversation was? Absolutely not, but your voice said, 'yes' or 'hi,' and I wasn't expecting you really even to be talking."

Katrina Cravy: "I feel like I called as soon as [Kim] told me. And I think I said, 'Is it OK for us to come?' And you were like, 'OK,' in a high-pitched tone. Still positive. Really positive."

Kim Buchanan: "We went to the hospital on Sunday. It took us a while to figure out how to get to her, right?"

She looked at Katrina at this point. They were about to meet Nuncie, the self-prescribed gatekeeper.

"And then we got to the ICU, and we didn't know if Nuncie was a friend or a nurse or a doctor or whatever. We really didn't. We were trying to peer into the room, and she wouldn't let us in."

We all laughed because of the sheer drama in Kim's voice as she recounted this story, especially since this is pretty funny to hear in hindsight.

Katrina Cravy: "And you know me, and Kim, too. As a journalist, not being able to get what you want and that there being somebody there that's telling you that you cannot go in."

The look of frustration on Katrina's face was palpable, as she remembered that day.

"And in my mind, it was like there was no hospital staff. It was just Nuncie."

We all laughed because now everybody knew that Nuncie is one of my sorority sisters.

"Like seriously. She met us at wherever it was and just said, 'I'm sorry, but she's not able to talk to anybody, and nobody's able to see her.' "

Kim Buchanan: "And we didn't know whether to believe her or not."

Katrina Cravy: "And she goes, 'We're not allowing anybody in.' And that was the thing that ruffled my feathers. Now looking back, I totally understand that they were totally protecting you."

Kim Buchanan: "Absolutely. They did the right thing."

Katrina Cravy: "I actually got mad, which is not normal protocol for me. Kim was the one who talked me down, which is usually the opposite."

We all broke out in laughter at the thought of Kim being the one to calm down the rest of us. But Katrina was frustrated. She did not know Nuncie and didn't trust that what she was saying was in my best interest.

Kim Buchanan: "And I'm like, 'Look, you and I have kids. We can't sit here 24 hours a day. There's a reason this woman is here, you know?' "

Katrina Cravy: "I recall Kim telling me, 'Vivian has to have these other friends. We are not able to be those people we were in the nineties. We are not there anymore.'"

Kim Buchanan: "Then I asked her, 'Well, do you want to sit here for 24 hours?' "

Katrina Cravy: "Well, no. I couldn't do that."

Kim Buchanan: "Exactly. So, we have to trust that this woman has the time, obviously, and that she knows what she's doing. We would do the same thing. We wouldn't want her to have this parade of visitors if she's really sick."

Katrina Cravy: "Kim was right. I had lost the argument."

Kim and Katrina decided to leave, but that's when people throughout the hospital started recognizing Katrina as a former TV personality. They adored Katrina and were stopping her to talk.

"And they want you to be you, and I'm pissed off now. My friend had a stroke. I don't know this woman. I can't see my friend."

That is when I chimed in. "All you had to do was tell them you had a rough day with Nuncie."

The laughter spilled from our table into the rest of the restaurant.

After Kim and Katrina tried to see me on Sunday, Susan decided to take a chance at visiting me on Monday.

Susan Kim: "I was prepared for Nuncie. And she was there, but so was your mom."

"I think my Mom must've let you in," I said.

Katrina Cravy: "Your mom would've let us in. Like if she would've seen us, it would've been OK. But we were like, we don't know this woman [Nuncie], and she doesn't know us. She's just doing what she's told."

Susan Kim: "But I did tell you the story about Nuncie. And you were laughing, and your Mom was laughing. It was funny."

Suddenly, I totally remembered the moment, one I hadn't thought about in five years. "When you walked in, the first thing you said was, '*Who is Nuncie?*'" I said. "And we all erupted in laughter, including Nuncie."

Susan remembered my talking a little bit during her visit, but it was early on, and I didn't quite have a real command of my speech at that point. The doctors were still monitoring me and giving me anti-swelling medicine for my brain. Mom and Nuncie did most of the talking with Susan during her visit.

Susan Kim: "One other thing, and I might be misremembering this too, but I feel like I knew this was happening. When I was visiting you, I feel like you got a delivery from the Bartolottas. Did that happen when I was there? All of a sudden, Jennifer Bartolotta came in with bags, like two fists of bags, filled with special food for you. Was that when I was there?"

This part is fuzzy to me, as well. However, I know that on a few occasions, some of my favorite local restaurants had food delivered to the hospital for my de facto caregivers and me.

Joe Bartolotta, a great Milwaukee chef, and his wife, Jennifer, owned several restaurants around the Milwaukee area, from French to steaks to seafood and everything in between. You are never disappointed at a Bartolotta restaurant. Plus, Joe accepted invitations from me to do food segments when

I worked for WTMJ-TV. I frequented his restaurants, and he was a good friend.

My other favorite restaurant at the time was Bosley on Brady. Michele Green (not to be confused with my soror, Michelle Greene) owned the Key-West-themed place famous for its shrimp and grits, seafood symphony and drinks introduced to us by the person I called the best bartender in the world, Jonathan Maye. But I have digressed.

Bartolotta's and Bosley delivered to us, one friend brought in Mason Street Grill, and another brought in sushi. Again, all of this is still fuzzy in my mind, but my mother and friends ate well. Apparently, I also enjoyed some of the non-hospital food fare, a small sign that I was turning a corner with my recovery.

One other sign that I was starting to get better was news that I would be going to rehab within the next week. Mom had left St. Louis so fast to come see about me that she needed to go back home to update Daddy and Grandma Louise, in addition to checking on their health. She didn't really want to leave me, but she felt comfortable that my circle of friends would handle the situation well. After all, somebody was always just in the waiting room, ready to give my mother a break or step in when anything was needed.

"When I was getting ready to leave, I told you what I was going to do," Mom said,

I did not really respond.

"Bye, honey," Mom said as she was about to head out the door. "I wish you could say, 'Bye, Mom.'"

That's when I looked up at her.

"Bye, Mom," I said.

"That nearly brought me to tears," Mom said as she recounted this story to me. "But I didn't want to cry in front of you."

She broke down in tears as soon as she left my room.

PART II

The Healing

CHAPTER EIGHT

Why Won't They Let Me Watch Modern Family?

One morning, I remember waking up, and I was in a room by myself. It was the room I would occupy for my remaining stay at the hospital. In my solitude, I remember picking up the remote control to see what was on television. The hospital cable offerings are not quite what you would find at home, but there were several stations that I could watch. Of course, I could watch the news on any of the local channels, but there was also TNT, one of my favorite networks, especially for an occasional rerun of *Law & Order*. The original version is my favorite, but I am not opposed to watching *SVU* or *Criminal*

Intent. I guess because it was the morning of a weekday, the only thing on TNT at the time was *Modern Family.*

Up until that point, I had not seen *Modern Family.* Several people I knew—and those I didn't—had raved about the show. Since no other shows interested me at that time, I decided that this was a good time to find out what I had been missing.

After the first episode, I was intrigued. I even chuckled a bit. You see, while I had lost the ability to talk, I could understand most things that were going on around me. I may not have been able to tell you about them, but I could definitely understand. So, with *Modern Family*, the characters—especially Cam— and the comedy, I found them all captivatingly hilarious. By the third episode, I was hooked. I ended up binge-watching the show throughout the rest of my stay at St. Luke's, finally understanding why this had become such a popular show.

I heard a knock. The door opened, and a nice nurse entered my room. She was very pleasant, like all the doctors and nurses with whom I had come in contact each day. However, this one shared with me news that meant I was about to be torn from my new favorite show. It was time for me to start a rigorous schedule of therapy.

I would undergo three types of therapy: occupational, physical, and speech. Having not endured a hospital stay quite like this one before, I had only a cursory knowledge of each. This was, unfortunately, my opportunity to become intimately acquainted with what each meant and why I had to participate to return to wellness.

Physical therapy (PT) is pretty self-explanatory. The stroke had left my right side limping, lagging, and weak. To transport me to various places, my caregivers used a wheelchair. We had to strengthen the right side of my body, so I had one session of physical therapy each day.

Since I could not talk, I had to start working on those skills. I had two sessions of speech therapy a day for the duration of my hospital stay. My doctors had no idea how long I would go without speaking, so my therapists were taking steps to teach me how to talk and write again. I remember speech therapists coming to my NICU room to begin that process, to no avail. Now I was in a private room, and my therapy sessions were crucial.

Finally, I had to undergo occupational therapy. Wikipedia, the popular, online encyclopedia, defines occupational therapy (OT) as "the use of assessment and intervention to develop, recover, or maintain the meaningful activities, or occupations of individuals, groups or communities." Basically, I had to begin relearning things that I had—up until that point—taken for granted, like how to get ready in the morning, go shopping in a manner that made sense or even cook a meal. My brain had to catch back up to my old life.

"Are you ready to get up, Vivian?" the nurse asked.

In my head, I said a sarcastic, *Not really. You see that I'm watching* Modern Family. *Can you come back?* However, I turned off the TV and complied. The woman was actually my occupational therapist. She began wheeling me out of my room and down the hall to a doorway that opened into what looked like a community shower - different shower stalls next to each other. These were larger-than-normal stalls, large enough to fit a bench and a second person.

My OT therapist had a bench in one of the stalls waiting for me. She helped me take off my hospital gown and helped me turn on the water, pointing out the soap and washcloth. She instructed me on how to wash myself. I remember it taking a little time, but we got through it, and she helped me put on new hospital garments. Then, back to my room we went.

When we rolled through the doorway of my room, June was there. I waved, and she greeted me as pleasant and friendly as ever, with a big smile. My occupational therapist told her we had one more task to complete, and then I could visit.

At that point, she instructed me to get out of the wheelchair and walk into my bathroom. It had a toilet, sink and shower, but the shower was much smaller than the one I had just left. She gave me a toothbrush and a small tube of toothpaste and told me to go ahead and brush my teeth. *Easy enough*, I thought. I squeezed some of the toothpaste onto the brush and put a little water on it, and I began brushing. I did sideways and up and down. I remembered that I had not done this for a while.

When I finished brushing, I leaned over the face bowl. Nothing happened. It's as if I expected something to happen but didn't quite know the next step, and if I was in control of it.

"Vivian, you have to spit it out," my therapist said firmly. "Come on, Vivian. You've got to spit."

I recalled thinking that I should have known that. I forced myself to empty the contents of my mouth and felt significantly inadequate. My therapist gave me a reassuring look, and I went back into my room to visit with June.

"My car automatically went to St. Luke's for a long time," said June. "Whenever I was on the expressway, it would automatically turn toward Holt Avenue, 27th Street and St. Luke's."

Overhearing the end of my OT session that day made June realize how tentative my situation still was.

"That bathroom-tooth-brushing thing was just really very disturbing to me," June said. "Because, when you think about it, those are motions that you automatically do, and you didn't know what to do."

My absolute favorite show during the time of my illness was *Scandal*, which aired every Thursday evening on ABC. It was a political thriller set in Washington, D.C., in the White House among all the aspects that make our nation's capital a place you either love or hate. (I happen to love D.C. and presidential shows and was looking for a good show to replace one of my original favorites, *The West Wing*.)

Scandal starred Kerry Washington as Olivia Pope, the ultimate "fixer" through her crisis management firm, Olivia Pope & Associates (OPA). However, this "fixer" was also having an affair with the President. *Scandal* was the first time in more than thirty years that a television show starred a black actress on a major television network (*Julia* starring Diahann Carroll was the other that aired in my lifetime, another favorite). Also, *Scandal* was the third show created by Shonda Rhimes, now one of the preeminent television producers and film writers in America.

When *Scandal* first hit the scene, I was mesmerized. It was definitely television I put on my calendar as an appointment, and I made *sure* that I was on my couch in front of the TV every Thursday night. I would literally be a bundle of nerves, balled up on my couch, almost afraid to breathe, from witnessing the fast-paced dialogue, murders, even torture, and extramarital affairs. The fall that I was in the hospital, *Scandal* was in its third season. A few of my sorors would sometimes come watch *Scandal* with me on Thursdays, but Beverly was my diehard *Scandal* partner. She always visited on Thursday. We would watch four episodes during my hospital stay.

"I don't think there was a day I didn't come down while you were in the hospital," Beverly said. "I wasn't working at the time, so I was available."

On Thursdays is when Beverly said my eyes *really* did the talking for me. "You couldn't talk, but when something happened, you would look at me [eyes wide] with a shocked look."

I remember wanting to talk about what I was seeing but not being able to give voice to my thoughts.

"You would get mad if a nurse came in and interrupted us," Bev said. "I would say, 'We're watching her favorite show,' and they would say, 'Oh, I will be really quick. It won't take but a second.' "

My stroke took away my memory and ability to speak, but my personality was still there. I was annoyed at the constant interruptions as I was watching my show. This would not happen at home.

One Thursday evening, Joan was sitting with me, and *Scandal* was just about to come on television. Nuncie and Beverly had not arrived yet, but the nurse had come in with my food.

"Do you want to eat before *Scandal*?" Joan asked.

"Yes," I said.

I was not answering in sentences at this time. I only replied in single words. Also, my friends were instructed not to feed me because my doctors wanted to see how well I could feed myself. However, my mother and friends were supposed to watch me to see if I was picking up the right utensils and maneuvering my fork or spoon correctly. They were charged with sharing their observations with my doctors.

"You had your food in front of you, and there was a dish of corn," Joan said. "So, I just sat there and watched you and then I said, 'Viv, what's that?'"

Joan was pointing to the corn. Joan said I looked at it and then looked at her. "I don't know what word to use," I said.

"It's corn," Joan said.

I repeated the word after her.

"But I'll never forget the look on your face," Joan said. She described a look of confusion. I knew what the corn was. I just didn't know what word to use. In my head, I would shut down when I did not have an answer to a question. Those were the frustrating times.

The name of my floor was 2-North. It was where the inpatient rehabilitation took place and where I spent twenty-two of my thirty-two days in the hospital. My everyday life there was routine, but each of my friends had a different story about that time period.

"I remember that they said we should be talking to you," said Joan. "So even though you weren't responsive, I'd talk about stuff, and Nuncie would talk about stuff. And then I said, 'I wonder if we should read her a book.' Then I said, 'Naw, she doesn't want to hear that. She wants to hear what's going on around the community.' "

Joan remembered the time a mutual acquaintance of ours strolled in and tried to look at my chart.

"Um, NO," said Joan. She grabbed my chart. The acquaintance tried to explain that she and her husband were concerned about me.

"I truly believe they were," said Joan. "I said, but no, you're not looking at her chart."

Joan also remembered not being there when I first opened my eyes in a conscious state. But she walked in one day, and I turned my head to look at her. A nurse was with me.

"Oh, my God! You're awake!" Joan screamed. "Vivie, you're awake!"

Joan said I did not smile. I just looked at her like I was trying to figure out who Joan was. She thought, *OK, she doesn't know me.*

"How do you feel?" Joan asked.

I blinked my eyes, and Joan thought, *maybe she can't talk.*

"Vivian, can you say good morning?" the nurse asked.

"Hi," I replied.

"Viv, do you know who I am?" Joan asked. "And you looked at me like I was crazy."

"Joan," I said, a bit perturbed at why she did not realize I knew who she was.

"Oh, OK," Joan said.

She remembered her and the nurse laughing at that moment. Another thing Joan remembered is when June baked me a pound cake. (She makes the best pound cakes.)

"June made a cake, cut it up in pieces, and put it in a brown paper bag," Joan said. "The idea was that when you woke up, we'd give you a piece every day."

The thought of this made us chuckle.

Jessica recalls, "Every day, we could see the progress once the bleeding stopped on the brain. Even when you couldn't talk, you were able to use your hands to communicate with us to let us know what you wanted or needed."

June would come up on her days and do activities with me. She always liked to take me on a walk through the hallways.

"You had to have a belt on to hold you just in case something happened," June said.

After one walk, June had brought supplies to polish my nails. "What color nails do you want?" June asked. "You said, 'red,' of course. So, I did your hands and your toes."

Even though I had lost my short-term memory, red has been my favorite color since childhood.

"We could tell by your eye recognition if you remembered or recalled stuff," Jessica said. "You never were in a stubborn mood or got frustrated with your situation. If you did, you would just kind of sit there and get quiet and just kinda nod your head or look at TV or something."

All my friends said that I was never mean-spirited or combative. I never turned my back to them. I seemed always to be willing to *try* to communicate, less so if I was tired.

"I was there one time when you were gone for therapy, and I waited 'til you and your mom came back," Jessica said. "You looked at me and smiled and waved. Your mom looked at me."

"She is exhausted," Mom said.

"I can tell," Jessica said. "I'm just going to sit here a little until she goes to sleep."

Once they put me to bed, I was asleep almost instantly.

"How long was she in therapy?" Jessica asked.

"She did two today, and they're coming back again this afternoon," replied Mom.

Everyone could tell that therapy took a lot out of me. My mother was the only person who went to my inpatient therapy sessions with me. She would report to my care circle what I had done each time. For a normal person, the activities were not a lot of work, but they were quite the task for someone who had suffered a massive stroke.

My speech and physical therapy sessions took place in the regular therapy area on 2-North. It was large enough to have several patients and therapists working at the same time, including three smaller offices for individual speech sessions and two conference rooms that could accommodate small groups. My occupational therapy involved field trips, which got me off my floor and even out into the surrounding neighborhood.

When we first arrived in my daily therapy room, all patients were taken to a central waiting area. It was not closed off, so we could still see the work that everyone else was doing. We just had to wait there until our therapist was ready for us. There was a similar waiting area for speech therapy, a table a little farther back and closer to the offices, but I never had my scheduled ST first. I always started with PT.

Still, all my therapists would try to encourage me to talk. They would greet me. Then I would return their greeting. They would then ask me what I had for breakfast that day. My routine was such that I would have just finished breakfast right before my first therapy session. My mind could remember what I had just eaten. My mouth just could not form the words to tell them. For the life of me, I could not understand why the words wouldn't form.

For PT, I would mostly exercise my weak leg with repetitive actions. There was a long stretch of the room with nothing impeding one's way, and that's where I would walk back and forth. In a matted area, right when you come in the door, there were aerobic steps and exercise balls for abdominal work. I was instructed to step up and down, over and over on those steps, in addition to doing several stretching exercises. Toward the end of my hospital stay, my PT therapist included an occasional squat.

The goal of my official speech therapy sessions was simply to restore my speech to the way it was pre-stroke. This included repeating words and comprehension exercises associated with the words. One time, I remember my therapist asking me to print my name. I did that easily. Then she told me to write down my home address. I began writing down the address and stopped mid-way during the second number of my con-dominium. I looked at my therapist in confusion.

"That's OK, Vivian," she said. "It will come back."

After my original OT session, when I relearned brush-ing my teeth, I grew to enjoy OT more. I think because the sessions got me off 2-North and into the hospital pharmacy. When we visited the pharmacy, my therapist gave me a list of items that I was supposed to purchase. We did this on three separate occasions. The activity was aimed at testing my organizational skills, whether my brain could put together sequences correctly. This activity was timed. Each time I got faster. My confidence was growing, and my inner competitive spirit was secretly celebrating.

My mother loved and appreciated all the attention my medical team paid me, but there is nothing like spiritual care. This is why probably her favorite place at Aurora St. Luke's Medical Center was the rooftop healing garden and conservatory. It is a 14,000 square-foot area on an eighth-floor rooftop in the mas-sive complex. It includes a 4,000 square-foot glass conservatory, which allows year-round access to the trees, shrubs, flowers, and a fountain in the garden. It also offers an expansive view of the Milwaukee skyline, including the Milwaukee Brewers' baseball stadium—Miller Park, downtown Milwaukee, and

Lake Michigan. Once I got better at therapy, Mom would visit in between sessions while I was resting.

"I prayed a lot and enjoyed the Healing Garden after you went into rehab," Mom said.

My mother also prayed a lot at the hospital chapel, which was in the same tower at St. Luke's as 2-North and my rehab room.

"Every time Marilyn and I would get there, we'd head straight to the chapel," Joan said. "And I thought I could pray, but Marilyn could pray. She was praying for a good forty minutes."

In addition to praying, my mother kept everybody in St. Louis abreast of my progress, and they were praying, too. Whether it was my father, my Grandma Louise, my mother's church or my mother's closest friends, I had prayer warriors in my corner.

"I talked to your Daddy every day," Mom said. "He would say, 'How's my baby?' every single time we talked."

The prayers seemed to be working. My doctors were finally telling everyone to expect me to make a 100% recovery, though it would still be a slow process.

CHAPTER NINE

God Flips a Switch

On the afternoon of Tuesday, November 19, after a full day of therapy sessions, I began actually forming sentences. It's hard to remember what triggered this enhanced speech exactly—perhaps it was the methodical exercises from each of my speech sessions—but I remember that my newfound ability just seemed to come out of nowhere. It is as if God flipped a switch and *poof,* I could talk again.

My mother was there and told me that it was probably time to give me back my iPhone. I had a landline in my hospital room, but my care team had unplugged it and carefully situated some of the flowers I had received in front of it. I never even noticed the phone in my room and never had the desire to use a phone anyway.

Mom mentioned a list of people who had called and who I might call back: Marlon, Raymond, and Tasha, to name a few. It was overwhelming to think that I had to call everybody back at once, especially with my therapy schedule. My mother said I could take my time and call them all back over the next several days. That's what I decided to do.

Mom wanted to bring me up to speed on my friend, Marlon. Dr. Marlon Moore is an oral and maxillofacial surgeon. We met when we both attended the University of Missouri-Columbia. We've been great friends ever since. His practice is in New York City. Over the years, I had often stayed with Marlon when I visited the Big Apple. In later years, his family grew to a wife and three children. I have stayed with the entire family before.

"Marlon called, and I thought he was calling about you," Mom said. "I answered when I saw his name pop up. I told him who I was, and he asked how you were. I told him you were still in ICU, thinking he had heard about your stroke. Then he told me he had not heard and was calling you because *he* was in ICU."

I was shocked. What were the chances of both of us, at the same age, never having true health problems, being in the hospital *and* in ICU? Marlon had gone to the doctor to see about some fatigue he was feeling. He ended up being admitted and was nursing a major heart issue, another story for another book.

After I had dinner that evening, Mom, Nuncie and I were watching a little TV when one of my church members and friends called wanting to visit. Mom told Julietta Henry that, of course, she could come visit.

"When I walked in the room, you said, 'Hello, Julietta,'" Julietta said.

She said I enunciated the 'Ts" just as I always did when I greeted her.

"I started dancing, I was so happy, 'cause I didn't know what to expect," Julietta said. "It's a miracle. She's alive. She's alive."

Julietta was afraid to come because of the announcement Pastor McVicker had made to the congregation two Sundays in a row. He had announced on the Sunday after I was hospitalized that I could not accept any visitors. He told them that he did not want anyone going to the hospital to see me because it was very serious.

"It was a shock," Julietta said. "I didn't know who was reporting back. People heard you had had a stroke, but no one knew how bad it was."

But Julietta was glad she took the risk of coming to see me because I could clearly communicate with her.

"Today is my first day speaking," I said, according to Julietta.

"And you knew who I was and everything," Julietta added.

Julietta even came bearing gifts. She brought some banana-nut bread she had made in her new bread maker for my mother. Mom was happy to take her snack back to my condominium with her that night.

After Mom left, I decided to call Raymond. Because of the two-hour time difference between the Central and Pacific time zones, it's always easier to call Raymond at night. I dialed his number.

"Hello," he answered.

"Hey, Raymond," I said.

"*Hey,*" he said.

His voice signaled that he was *clearly* happy to hear from me and actually surprised.

"You can talk," he said.

Neither one of us can remember exactly what was said during that initial phone conversation, but Raymond remembered one thing.

"You called as though nothing happened," Raymond said. "It threw me for a loop."

From that point on, I talked to Raymond every day. He told me that so many people were concerned and expressing it on Facebook that he decided to "like" things on Facebook that he thought I would "like."

"You're such a popular person. Everybody was vested in your well-being," Raymond said. "I couldn't be there. That was my way of being there."

Raymond also helped me keep some of my frequent flier miles. I was scheduled to go to Dallas on November 1, 2013, to visit a soror and see the Green Bay Packers play the Dallas Cowboys in their new football stadium. Clearly, I could not make it, so Raymond began calling all the airlines and giving my name to find out if they had a reservation for me. He finally lucked out with Delta Airlines but had to pretend he was my husband to get the information.

"That's my wife. She had a situation and can't take the flight," Raymond told the Delta Airline representative.

You might say this was the closest Raymond and I ever got to being married.

"Being your partner at the time, I took that as my job," Raymond said to me.

Fortunately, I was able to use those Delta SkyMiles at a later date. Raymond and I did not talk long that first night. After we hung up, I finally fell asleep after an exciting day in my recovery.

I am naturally an early riser. I am much more alert and high functioning in the mornings, even if I don't like to be out and about to go to a Girl Scouts breakfast. I woke up around 5 a.m. on the morning of Wednesday, November 20. It was dark in my room, but I remembered my phone. I picked it up and decided to go onto Facebook, my favorite social media site. My "Timeline" was lit up with messages of surprise and well-wishes from the previous twenty-six days. I was overwhelmed. There were literally hundreds of messages. I began reading them. After a while, I started "liking" them. A producer I used to work with responded to my actions by posting, "I saw that 'like' on Facebook, Viv. I'm taking it as a sign that you're getting better." I decided to not respond to him. I just wasn't quite ready, knowing that I did not have the energy to respond to all my friends on Facebook.

The next thing I knew, I received a text message from my friend and soror, Tressa Williams. Her first name is pronounced with the long "e" as in Tree-sa (it annoys me when people mispronounce her name, although she takes it in stride and never corrects them). It was a similar message.

"Is that really you liking things?" Tressa texted.

"Yes," I texted back.

"Can you talk?" Tressa texted.

"Yes," I texted back.

The phone rang. It was Tressa.

Tressa was so happy to hear my voice. She expressed how worried she was and said she and her husband, Ken, had been praying for my recovery. Tressa and Ken live in California, and Ken is a pastor. I have known Tressa a long time—since I pledged Delta Sigma Theta. We roomed in college my senior year when she was starting her career with State Farm Insurance. I was even in Tressa's and Ken's wedding. We talked for a brief period of time before hanging up.

I still had energy, so I went ahead and reached out to Tasha Sledge, the third caller Mom had mentioned. Tasha is a soror and stepped in when I asked her to serve as secretary of the Milwaukee Alumnae Chapter of Delta Sigma Theta when the elected secretary had to resign after being offered a job out of the state. Tasha revolutionized taking minutes back then by using her laptop. She later became chapter president, and we served as co-chairs of our Founders Day luncheon after that when another president asked us to serve together. We used to joke that she was HR (Human Resources), and I was PR (Public Relations), and that's how we ran our committee. From those days, I know that Tasha is an early riser as well, so I knew she would be up to take my call.

"Tasha," I said when she answered. "This is Vivian."

"What!" Tasha exclaimed. "I can't believe this. I have been so worried about you and praying for you."

"Thank you," I said. "My mom told me that you called."

"I had seen these messages on Facebook," Tasha said. "Then I called your phone and talked to your mother, and she told me what happened."

"I know," I said. "She told me."

"Then I talked to Beverly, and she's been keeping me up to date," Tasha said.

Suddenly, I sensed tears as Tasha's voice became shaky over the phone.

"Tasha, are you crying?" I asked. "Why are you crying? I'm OK."

Tasha is very caring, but she is no-nonsense and always in control of her emotions, so this shakiness surprised me.

"I just couldn't think of you not being able to talk again," Tasha said. "Praise God. Praise God! You can talk."

We did not talk much longer because Tasha had to get ready for work, and I had to get ready for my day of therapy. I got up and got ready for the day. Mom showed up, her normal routine—however, this time, she brought with her several sweatsuits. I put on one of them, and we waited for one of the transporters to get me.

My first therapy session was scheduled for 9:30 a.m. Someone was always there to wheel me to the therapy area, usually about ten minutes before my session. It was about 9:28 a.m., and I was getting impatient. This is one of my mother's favorite memories.

"The guy had not come to get you, and we started walking," Mom said. "We met him mid-way, and he said, 'What are you trying to do, take my job?' You told him that you didn't want to be late."

I guess Mom likes that memory because it clearly signaled that I was getting back to myself. I did not need the wheelchair, and I could clearly state to the transporter why I had made the decision to walk on my own.

I had something new on my schedule one day—an on-site meeting with a support group. It was the last appointment on my calendar. We followed the hallway to the room, winding our way through the hospital. There were already people in the room, sitting around a table. We all waited quietly until a woman came in to lead the discussion. As I sat around the table, listening to the other patients in the group, I could not help but wonder *why am I here?* These people were having trouble speaking.

There was an older woman who I had seen in the hospital who could talk clearly, but she had shared that she had worked for a local bank when she suffered a brain aneurysm. The impact of her illness would prevent her from going back to work. Her mind just wouldn't let her do the calculations she once needed for her job. This was the first time I began to wonder if I would be able to return to my job and what I would do if I couldn't.

An older man was having trouble forming his words. We could understand him, but he spoke very slowly and deliberately. I found myself on the edge of my seat, leaning in, anticipating the next word in his sentence.

There was a young woman, considerably younger than me. I think she was about 29. She could not really form words at all, but she had been out of the hospital for years. She wrote her answers to the questions asked of her in the group and then showed us what she had written.

Finally, the group leader looked at my mother and me, almost signaling to us that it was our turn to speak. Apparently, we were the newest people in this group.

"My name is Marilyn King, and this is my daughter, Vivian," my mother said. "Vivian suffered a stroke on October 25th, and she has been here in the hospital since that day."

Everyone greeted us. I stayed silent. I was so confused because I had just started talking the day before. I felt like I had nothing in common with these people.

"Vivian could not speak when she first got here," Mom said. "But miraculously, she began speaking just yesterday."

The crowd clapped. The group leader explained that aphasia comes in different forms. One dictionary described it as "the loss of a previously held ability to speak or understand spoken or written language, due to disease or injury of the brain." She explained that this is why everyone in our circle experienced aphasia in his or her own unique way. The discussion incorporated questions from some of the people in the room, asking about ways to improve, others in the circle offering advice, and an announcement of other groups at various times at a variety of locations. The woman from the bank attended all the groups at times.

In the center of the table, there were purple wristbands with the words, "Living with Aphasia" printed on them, along with brochures with more information. At the end of the hour-long session, I concluded that I must have aphasia and that this information ultimately would help me. Embracing that thought fully, I picked up one of the wristbands and a brochure.

That evening, Katrina came to visit me. She had called my mother to get permission. My mother obliged because I was finally talking. Katrina was the first one of the TV Sisterhood to visit after I started talking. She was surprised, considering the condition I had been in early on and was cautious about wanting to push my speaking skills too far. But I explained to her that it was OK, that it was as if God had flipped a switch and I could talk again.

"We watched TV, talked to your Mom and that's how I learned about the police officer showing up," Katrina said.

My mother shared the details of how she first heard about my stroke, how Joan got in touch with her through the University City Police Department.

"And we were talking about customer service and different nurses who were coming in," Katrina said. "And you were saying that's a good one."

As I talked to her, I was pointing out the nurses that I really liked best as they would come in to check on me or give me my dinner.

"You were saying really cool things," Katrina said. "You were saying 'Working for a hospital, I have learned so much from the patient aspect of this. I see how certain people have a good bedside manner, and others don't. You were looking at what kind of customer service you were getting. You were saying, 'I have surveys.' You were gaining this knowledge. I remember that for sure."

We then talked about how my doctors said I was relatively young to have a stroke. Sure, there are people younger than me who have had a stroke. But because I was active, only 49, and received immediate medical attention since I was at a public event, all of that contributed to my recovering pretty quickly.

"Didn't they also say that you were above-average intelligence?" Katrina asked.

"They *did* say that!" I responded, surprised that this memory came rushing back as I was talking to Katrina.

"Let's not forget about that," Katrina said. "Because I remember in a funny way, you told me, 'They say I'm recovering fast because I was pretty smart.' And I remember going, 'Yes, you are.' "

"I can't believe I said that to you," I said, laughing.

"You did, and it was hilarious," Katrina said. "When you're good friends, you can say something like that."

"I had forgotten about that," I said.

"That was one of the reasons they thought you were conquering all the rehab," Katrina said. "if I remember correctly, they had given you blocks of times for you to get to this point and then the next point, and you were getting there faster than they thought."

Katrina's visit was so timely and such a breath of fresh air. At that moment, we had no idea that I would be getting out of the hospital soon.

Now that I could finally talk and express myself, my mind started racing and thinking about all the things I was involved in and missing. I was Milwaukee Urban League Board Chair at the time, and before my stroke, we were planning the 54th Annual Equal Opportunity Day Luncheon. The event celebrates diversity and features awards to community members and a keynote speaker who talks on an economic theme. It was scheduled for the next day, Thursday, November 21, and I had been the one to help secure Paula Williams Madison, a former journalist, television executive, and now a businesswoman who is CEO of her family's investment group and a media consulting firm. Madison is also a member of Delta Sigma Theta. I had so much vested in this event, and here I was in the hospital.

The wheels in my brain really started turning as I sat in solitude after my mother and Katrina went home. Could I somehow make the luncheon tomorrow? After all, I could now talk and adequately greet people. All I'm doing is laying in this bed, except for when I have to go to therapy. I feel fine. I could pretend to go for a walk around the hospital, have one of my friends pick me up, swing by my place to get me something appropriate to wear, and then slip into the Pfister Hotel just to see one of my idols speak and say 'hello.' My body became exhilarated at the thought.

Then my logical brain took over. What kind of chaos might this cause? Nobody had seen me since my collapse at the Girl Scouts breakfast, and they would be surprised and wanting to ask questions. This might take away from Paula's speech. Plus, which one of my friends would really help me sneak out of the hospital? Not being able to think of one who would go along with this plan, I thought better of it. In the hospital I stayed.

On Saturday, November 23, my friend, Shawn Taylor, came to visit. Shawn majored in journalism with me at the University of Missouri-Columbia. She was a news editor and columnist at the Chicago Tribune until she left and founded her own communications, media and marketing firm called Treetop Publishing. Shawn drove up to Milwaukee from Chicago that morning and was just in the middle of our visit when my occupational therapist came in. We were going on another field trip. My therapist invited Shawn to come along, and we all put on our coats and headed to Starbucks, which was right across the street from the hospital.

I was instructed to stand in line, order, and complete the transaction at the cash register. Again, these tasks may sound painfully simple, but I had had a major brain injury. These were important building blocks for my recovery. They were all happy with my performance on this day. We had a millennial at the register, and he could not figure out the change. Since math has always been one of my strong suits, I offered the correct amount. He thanked me for it, and my therapist was pleased.

On subsequent days, we went to Walmart to test my thought process when shopping at such a huge store. We also did an indoor activity at a built-in apartment at St. Luke's. I had to navigate the kitchen. I ended up making grilled-cheese sandwiches. Mom was such a trooper. She ate her sandwich for her dinner that night, at least in front of me.

CHAPTER TEN

Goodbye, Condo South!

Jokingly, I now call Aurora St. Luke's Medical Center my "condo south." After all, I spent more than a month there, and it all began on the day I collapsed at the Girl Scouts breakfast. But good news came on Monday, November 25. My rehab doctor came into my room during his morning rounds and told me I was going to be able to leave the hospital the *next day*. I still had a full day of therapy sessions, including one more field trip to Walmart, but all my therapists agreed that I did not have to stay at the hospital for the additional therapy I needed. I could now be helped through outpatient therapy and navigate from home.

Thus, the day was full of anticipation. I started gathering all the things my mother and "sisters" had brought to the hospital, getting them ready to take back home. We spoke with my doctor about what I needed when I got home. I definitely needed someone to drive me to my appointments because when you have a seizure, state law prohibits you from driving for at least ninety days. I also needed someone to watch me around the house. Mom needed to take another trip back to St. Louis to check on my father and grandmother, so the plan was for me to stay with June.

There was some talk about my going to St. Louis for a while, but I nixed that idea. It would've been easier for Mom since she was already a caretaker for my father and grandmother, but I felt instantly uncomfortable. I would've had to find therapists to work with me. I'm not saying there is anything wrong with health care in St. Louis, but I was so used to my own health care system that I got a sinking feeling in my stomach every time I thought about having to leave my familiar surroundings. I ended up talking to June about it, and that's when she gladly offered for me to stay at her place.

Finally, November 26 arrived, and it was time for me to say goodbye officially to my condo south. It was two days before Thanksgiving, and I could not think of a better time to leave. I was so thankful. My doctors told me I was way ahead of schedule. They had set a date of Thursday, December 5, 2013, for my leaving the hospital, based on my condition when I entered the hospital, but I had blown through all my therapy milestones and was being allowed to leave nine days early.

I had strict instructions. Everything was noted in my discharge papers. I must admit that reading and fully understanding them was overwhelming, and I feel that I'm reasonably intelligent. I don't know if it was the format, the fact that all of my follow-up appointments seemed to be scattered around the city or that I had just suffered a stroke and was not completely healed. Whatever it was—or if it was a combination—I can't imagine people who struggle with reading or grasping everyday life being fully able to comprehend or manage what doctors expect of patients. Bottom line: We all need help. I was so grateful for my tribe.

My doctor told me that he recommended me going to Aurora West Allis Medical Center for my outpatient therapy because they have an excellent reputation. It sounded good to me! He said he could have one of his nurses set up my first appointment, but all the locations and numbers were listed on my discharge papers, and I could make the appointments myself. Of course, I jumped at the chance to have them do it. He said I could start as early as that week, or if I wanted, I could take Thanksgiving off and start the following week. I needed a break, so I asked them to make the appointments starting after Thanksgiving.

My doctor then asked me if I had a primary care physician. I hated to admit that I did not, per se. I had an OB/GYN to take care of my reproductive system, my mammograms, etc., but I did not have an official primary care physician. He said one of my appointments needed to be with my primary care physician. He then mentioned that he had a good friend who was an excellent internist and was building her practice, Dr. Madhu Gupta. I ended up being scheduled to see her that next Monday.

While I had been in the hospital, one of the things the doctors did was monitor my blood thickness. The goal was to keep my blood thin enough to prevent future clots. Thus, I was on what's called warfarin or Coumadin˚. I would need to continue taking this blood thinner post-hospital. In fact, I would have a weekly appointment to test my blood. I could go to another location or visit the Anti-Coagulation Clinic at St. Luke's. By then, I felt comfortable at my condo south. St. Luke's it was.

I would also need a follow-up appointment with my rehab specialist in about two to three weeks, and I would need one with my neurologist, whom I didn't really know at that point. In all, I had to see six different people among doctors, specialists and therapists.

Finally, my doctor asked me if I had any questions. With Raymond in the back of my mind and thinking of my habits pre-stroke, I asked the doctor about when I could resume taking birth control pills. He got the most shocking look on his face.

"Oh, no," he said. "You won't be taking birth control pills anymore. They are what led to your stroke."

My mother was in the room. I looked at her and then looked back at him.

"What?" I asked.

"You will not be taking birth control pills anymore," he said.

He then promised that we would talk later but said he had to continue his rounds. Once he walked out of my room, I turned to my mother.

"Did you know this?" I asked.

"Yes," she said.

"Does Daddy know?" I asked.

"Yes," she said.

Can you say *embarrassed?* I was 49, of course, but I had never really discussed my sex life with my parents, especially my father. Oh, well, I guess "the cat's out of the bag" as they say. I have had sex. I chuckle at the thought of an unmarried 49-year-old having this fact revealed to her parents.

The wait to leave the hospital felt like a long one, perhaps because I was anxious. I thought I was going to be discharged in the morning, but the time stretched on into the afternoon. Many of my hospital caregivers used that time to check on me but also to say their goodbyes.

There was a knock at my door. It was a woman I did not recognize. My mother and I both said hello, but Mom seemed more familiar with the woman.

"When I heard you were leaving, I had to come see for myself," the woman said. "I was your speech therapist when you were in ICU."

"Oh," I said. "You saw me when I was a *mess*."

We all laughed a little.

"You were struggling," the woman said. "But what a blessing to see you now."

I was struck by the fact that she used the word "blessing."

"Do you mind if we pray?" she asked.

"No, not at all," Mom and I both said, almost simultaneously.

We bowed our heads, and she said a prayer for me. I was awestruck. In such a scientific setting, I knew my tribe had faith, but I had not thought about the lives my caregivers lead when they leave their jobs.

The speech therapist wasn't the only one. My favorite occupational therapist had gotten transferred to another floor during my stay, so I had not seen her for a couple of weeks. I was thrilled to see her when she decided to stop by. Again, she had heard during one of their meetings that this was my last day. Mom and I could not thank her enough for all her work with me.

"You must have thought I was crazy when you had to tell me to spit out my saliva when I was brushing my teeth for the first time," I said.

"You remember that?" she replied.

"Yes," I said.

"Well, you have come a long way," she said, "and I wish you the best."

"Thank you," I said.

"Do you mind if I say a prayer?" she asked.

"Of course, not," I responded.

This time, she, Mom, and I held hands in a small circle as she prayed for my continued recovery. When she left, I marveled again at the juxtaposition between spirituality and science, and from a caregiver's perspective. I really felt truly blessed that some of my caregivers exhibited such faith. I was equally surprised that they wanted to say goodbye to me.

"Each therapist loved you dearly," Mom said.

When it was finally time to leave St. Luke's, I could not have been happier. Neither could Mom.

"I was ecstatic upon discharge. I had been there every day and had seen your progress," Mom said. "I thanked the Lord over and over again. You had made a miraculous recovery."

June drove us to my home so Mom could pack for her trip to St. Louis, and I could switch out things I did not need over the next week for things I *would* need. She and Joan had previously straightened up my room, and I was grateful because I had been so busy that my closets looked like a *disaster zone*. We finished there and then traveled to June's condominium. I settled into what would be my room for the next week. We grabbed a quick bite to eat and then took Mom to the airport.

"When I left at Thanksgiving, I really didn't want to leave," Mom said. "I knew June would take good care of you, so I didn't feel quite so bad."

We hugged, and then Mom was off to St. Louis.

CHAPTER ELEVEN

The Road Back to Work

June has such a lovely home. Every time I visit, it makes me happy to be surrounded by such beauty. She has exquisite taste, which extends to her decor. However, what always made my time at June's even more special is the love that's palpable every time you walk across the threshold of her condominium. I was so glad to be staying in Milwaukee with her and Bill, while Mom traveled back to St. Louis to check on my father and grandmother.

I was glad to have a break from my therapy sessions, but I also recognized the importance of trying to help my progress in their absence. I wanted to see for myself if my brain would help me write, so I began keeping a journal. What follows are excerpts. Please note that some names have been changed to protect individual privacy.

Post-Hospital: Day 1

(Tuesday, Nov. 26, 2013)

Tonight was the first night I spent outside St. Luke's Medical Center. My mother went home, and I am at June's house. It is absolutely wonderful. For dinner, June made Bill and me short ribs, rice with gravy, haricot verts [green beans in French], and South Carolina tomatoes. (June is a South Carolina native.) Everything was fabulous. I always knew that there was a God, but the love and peace I got from St. Luke's, my family, my sorors, my friends and beyond proves it.

Post-Hospital: Day 2

(Wednesday, Nov. 27, 2013)

Day 2 was an extremely busy day. We had two very important appointments. First, my nail appointment. Second, my hair appointment. :-) You always know you're doing better when you want to make sure you look your best.

The first person I saw outside my close circle of friends was Dana. I can't remember her last name, but she does etiquette. She gave me such a warm, wonderful hug. There was no pressure, just blessings coming from her that made me feel good. The other blessed aspect of my nail appointment was the fact that my favorite nail person was working that day. She had temporarily left to go work in Minnesota. It was so good to see her and have her as my first appointment. She shared with me that her father recently had a stroke and that it ruined her mother's visit with her.

Finally, you never know how an event affects you until you hear an account from someone else's perspective. My journey to get my hair done was so astonishing. My stylist, Ivory, was not at the event where I had my stroke, but she knew many people there. She told me that my incident disrupted the entire setting. I had fallen out on the table, they called the paramedics and then asked if there was a doctor in the house.

Genyne called my friend, June, and asked her to meet at the hospital. They were taking me to Aurora Sinai. June met me there, having told the Emergency Room people that she was my sister. She was there when I was initially answering questions. The funniest part was that they asked me if I could be pregnant. I told them, "yes." Not! :-)

Anyway, June says we were at Sinai for about an hour when they said I needed to go to St. Luke's. I was there for 32 days. For three weeks, I could not talk. Some people would call that a blessing. :-) Now I can talk enough to tell you that the Girl Scouts breakfast resumed. :-)

Post-Hospital: Day 3

(Thursday, Nov. 28, 2013—Thanksgiving)

Day 3 outside of the hospital was Thanksgiving. I spent it at June's house. Not only did I help June make the pound cake, but I made two sweet potato pies myself. I found two recipes to review online. Then I finally caught up with my godmother, Aunt Joyce. She used to make us two sweet potato pies for Thanksgiving and Christmas. Some health issues kept her from doing this over the past three years. We combined her thoughts with my favorite of the two online recipes and voila, two fantastic pies.

I go on to write, in detail, about the rest of the food, and how June had all our guests go around the table to share why we were thankful that Thanksgiving. What struck me with these first few excerpts is that each day, I had more stamina and more organization in my thoughts. My journal writing was starting to do what I had hoped it would do. The next few excerpts reveal how I am slowly learning more about my ordeal, and my thoughts are turning to the future.

Post-Hospital: Day 4

(Friday, Nov. 29, 2013)

What can you say about the day after Thanksgiving except left-overs, leftovers, leftovers? I had pound cake and my first ever sweet potato pie that I made for lunch. (I know. Not healthy.) Then I had turkey, orzo salad, yams and greens for dinner. Bottom line: the day after Thanksgiving was great. In fact, absolutely delicious.

The most interesting part of the day came from two visitors I received. The first guest was Gerald, an old friend I used to date. The second guest was Roger, who used to do my hair. Gerald has loved me for a little while, not sure how long. Plus, he lives in the same building where June lives. Fortunately, he abided by the rules set by June [about visiting.] However, we decided to let him come over so that he could have a chance to see me.

It is, again, always fascinating to find out how much people seem to care about you. Gerald talked about how glad he was that we were able to have the conversation we were having. He talked about how wonderful June was in keeping people away from me, saying that he launches into a protective mode because of it. He told me how he was ready to accept whatever was happening but that this was unfair. He told me how I was a gift.

He also told me that he believes he was a confidante of June, and at their last meeting, she felt comfortable showing how my ordeal was affecting her. He believes June was preparing him, just in case. I look at Gerald as a buffer for my second guest.

Roger was supposed to stop by at 5:30 p.m., but he fell asleep and was a little late. It's just as well. I had babysitters for each moment of the time June and Bill were out on a date night. Roger is suffering from cancer. We went to visit him the Sunday before the episode that landed me into the hospital. Bev and I needed to see Roger. At first glance, he did not seem as sick as we knew he was. He was undergoing chemotherapy right in his bed. He was in good spirits. He had snacks for his visitors. We took him a couple of "Get Well Soon" balloons, in addition to candy.

Roger and I believe that there is a reason we both went through these health issues, especially at the same time. For me, I needed a break. I think God said he was going to do something drastic to put me on the right track. That drastic move was the stroke I had that resulted in a mild case of aphasia. For three weeks, my brain was covered in blood. The left side of my brain was affected. This meant that my right side had some complications. For instance, I initially had to be transported in a wheelchair at the hospital. Shortly before I started talking, more than a week before I was let out early, I began walking to my therapy sessions. I was supposed to be let out on Thursday, December 5. I left the hospital on Tuesday, November 26, two days before Thanksgiving.

This departure is giving me a chance to reflect. I will have time to right my course. I will have time to clean my closets, throw away junk I don't need and get my life back in order. Ironically, I will also have time to write, which is what I am doing now. My musical is next.

For Roger, I am hoping his high spirits mean that he will be around for a long time. He just finished working on a musical, The Book of Mormon. I think this timing put him in the position of having the insurance he needed to handle this health issue. I believe that Roger and I have the right tools and connections to get this done. I will keep you posted.

Post-Hospital: Day 5

(Saturday, Nov. 30, 2013)

The weekends are great for visiting. After waking up late, I read my Bible, talked to Raymond, and got up to get ready for Cecelia, Tracey and Beverly to stop by June's house to see me. Cecelia and Tracey arrived at around the same time. Tracey brought me thank you notes, shower gel, lotion and Nair. Cecelia brought me white roses. All were much appreciated.

The most interesting part of the visit was our conversation. We laughed, we talked, caught up with everything that was going on with the people in our lives. We talked about Cecelia's travels with her husband, Randy. We talked about Tracey's psychology education and the new man in her life. We talked about my illness and the man in my life. It was just good to laugh and be in the presence of positive people who care about you.

Before Tracey and Cecelia left, June started dinner. We had beef tenderloin, kale salad, fresh tomatoes from South Carolina and haricot verts. It almost made Tracey turn to eating beef. :-)

Once Cecelia and Tracey had gone, it was Beverly's turn to visit. She had the dinner shift this evening. She was floored by June's dinner. She enjoyed every morsel. Then it was time to get the latest on the sorority. Kim is doing a great job as chapter president. Our chapter has already done more public service in three months than it did in the past two years. I am proud of her. We also talked about Bev's new job. She is a recruiter for Bryant and Stratton. She received valuable experience in this area from UWM. Her new boss wants her to study and tutor with him. She seems excited. I am extremely happy.

As I close this day, it is appropriate to note that all of us single women need to get our houses in order. We need to have everyone's info on emergency contacts, etc. We must work on that soon.

Post-Hospital: Day 6

(Sunday, Dec. 1, 2013)

A look back at Sunday shows nothing but blessings. It began with Tracey picking me up for church. I thought this visit would be overwhelming, but it was anything but that. We eased in just after the 8 a.m. service started. It didn't seem that crowded. By the end of the morning, there were more people in the service, but we figured a lot of people were out of town for the holidays.

Slowly people began noticing me. Then I waved at Pastor when he came in. I had already texted him to let him know I was headed to church. He seemed to like my wave. Then Pastor got up to preach. He mentioned that it was a good day because I was there. That made me feel good. :-)

After church, Pastor invited Tracey and me to eat breakfast with him and his family. We did. It was nice. His son, Wesley, was there and had not heard of my illness until recently. We talked about his traveling and his helping with my musical. He wants to move to Las Vegas to work on scores and jingles. He said he'd help. Soon it was time to leave. June and I decided to make brunch plans for noon. So, when Tracey dropped me off, we decided to pick a place. We picked the brunch at Blue Jacket.

It was absolutely fabulous. I had the pork shoulder hash. She had the grilled pork chop hash, and Bill had the French toast. I treated. After brunch, we made our way to Lela, just to check in on Tracey. It was fun to be in the shop, even if I had no plans to buy something. It was just good to be amongst the living and enjoying what they were.

Finally, we arrived back home. I set up to begin writing thank you notes. However, I was distracted by the television, Juju baby, aka Jace, and conversation. At least, I sorted them by work, family, general friends, sorors, multiples and flowers. I received about ninety physical acknowledgments. I wrote only ten thank you notes. Yikes! The process of getting back online after I mail my thank you notes has been officially delayed. Still, God is good.

Post-Hospital: Day 7

(Monday, Dec. 2, 2013)

You might call it the slow reveal. Each day, I learn something new about the extent of my illness. My day began with an appointment at the anti-coagulation office. They tested my blood. It was only 1.8, pretty thick and susceptible to clots. It's supposed to be between 3.0 and 3.5. This means I have to take more Coumadin to make my blood a little thinner.

My next stop on Monday was to my primary care physician, Dr. Madhu Gupta. She is really cute and nice. She's the one who finally told me that I had a blood clot, which led to a stroke, which ultimately led to the seizure I had at the Girl Scouts breakfast on October 25. She then shared with me that they can't exactly pinpoint why I had my stroke, but it is likely birth control pills. At my age, in my late forties, I should not be taking them because they can cause blood clots.

Dr. Gupta also mentioned that I had sinus thrombosis. So, I must have had this issue for quite some time. Looking back, I think it has been building up for years, probably about two, to be exact. I should have gone to the doctor to see about my sinus troubles. By the way, I do like my doctor.

Post Hospital: Day 8

(Tuesday, Dec. 3, 2013)

Tuesday was my day to head home finally. Susan was picking my mother up from the airport and then swinging back to June's house to pick me up. While I could stay at June's forever, it was good to be finally getting back home.

Susan is very much the encourager, so she believes (and so do I) that this is going to be my first book. Thus, she is busy snapping pictures of my saying goodbye to June and Bill and gathering all my things. She is such a caring person. I love her.

Once we arrived home, our next gift was from Kim, Rick, Katrina, and Susan. Katrina first came over with bags of groceries for us. She had everything on my list: salmon, catfish, ground chuck, apples, grapes, California cuties, orange juice, grapefruit juice, cereal, milk, eggs, sweet potatoes, crust, water, etc. We had enough food for at least a week.

Later in the afternoon, I get this call from downstairs. It's a person who says he is Rick with a delivery. I tell him to come on up. Then I tell my mother what the person said. She replies, "Kim's Rick?" To which I said, 'now that you mention it, he did sound like Rick.' LOL. Can you say, 'Duh?' I'll be glad when this brain injury aftermath is over. Geez.

Our first meal was spinach salad. It was delicious. Then it was time to get ready for my second official outing, an evening with Harry Belafonte.

Mr. Belafonte is 87 years old and STILL fine. Most importantly, he has a lot to say about this world and his "space" in it. He has long been a Civil Rights advocate, in addition to an accomplished actor. He talked about being called by Dr. Martin Luther King, Jr. and marching with him. He talked about having a conversation with Jamie Foxx, who admitted that he "didn't know shit." Jamie was petitioning Harry to fill him with knowledge.

The format of the evening was very conducive to having a conversation with Harry and not just hearing a speech, if you will. I believe the emcee is an anchor at CBS 58. She did a nice job.

The best part about the evening was an unexpected gift. We were too late to stand in line to buy a book that Harry wrote, but we found an angel in Kim Montgomery's former co-worker in the Mayor's office. Forgive me because I can't remember her name right now. I will have to ask Kim. Anyway, they had gotten books just before the program started. Right before it ended, this woman ducked out so that she could be the first in line to get her book signed. After the program, I was talking to Kim when this woman walks up. Kim introduced us and we began talking about how wonderful Harry Belafonte was. That's when I mentioned that I wished I could've gotten a book to get it signed by Harry. Lo and behold, the woman hands me her book. She said that she was touched by what I had gone through and wanted me to have it. I tried not to take it, but she insisted. What a major blessing!

Post-Hospital: Day 9

(Wednesday, Dec. 4, 2013)

Wednesday was an early day for Mom and me and a busy day. We were up bright and early to take my car to get serviced. We left the house at about 7:40 a.m. to get to Andrew Toyota. We were the third car at the shop, early enough to get the first ride home.

The journal ends there. Admittedly, it is incomplete. I can tell that I had other things to write because I had notes corresponding to dates through December 11. For instance, on this last entry, I had notes about our going to see the movie, *Best Man Holiday*, with Tracey, and providing lunch for 2-North, the floor at St. Luke's where I spent the most time. The notes also list my anti-coagulation visits on later days, Christmas shopping, therapy at West Allis, and my first time back at a sorority meeting on Saturday, December 7, and church again on Sunday, December 8.

On my first day, I could really only write one paragraph. I remember thinking at the time that this was all I could do, but each day got better. I was, indeed, on the path to healing and on the road back to work.

CHAPTER TWELVE

Social Media Can Be Social

Some people call Facebook the devil. For me, Facebook was a blessing during my health ordeal. It was how many of my friends found out that I was in trouble, and it is how many of them expressed their concern. There were literally hundreds of messages from childhood, high school, and college friends to sorority sisters and colleagues. Here is just a fraction of the outreach.

Troy

"Good morning to all my DST friends. A practically lifelong friend of mine, Ms. Vivian King, is recovering from an illness. Though you may not know her, she's a beloved spark of energy and could use your prayers. So, I'm asking each of

WHEN THE WORDS SUDDENLY STOPPED

you, and any other Deltas who don't know her, to introduce yourselves by dropping her a line via FB. It would be greatly appreciated. #smooches"

Annette

"Hi, Vivian – I recently learned on Facebook that you are not well due to a health issue. Wow, what a surprise! I miss your enthusiastic & fun posts of your travels, people & events. I wish you a speedy recovery. I will keep you in my prayers. May God's healing powers be with you right now."

Stephanie

"Get well soon. Without you out and about, the fashion bar in Milwaukee is lowering, and we are all beginning to wear pants with stretchy waistbands. ☺"

Carol

"Stopped by after realizing that I haven't seen any activity from you! What the? You not trying to be sick on me? *I'm not havin it*!!!"

Polly

"Good morning from Colorado.
I'm thinking of you and your
entire posse this morning."

Eugene

"Thankful to see some "likes" posted from the one and only Vivian King. That really makes it a great holiday!"

Melissa

"So happy to see you are getting better! And amazing to see all the lives you have touched as we get to read all the prayers, well wishes and humor. I guess it's times like these when you really find out how much people care about you. But don't do it again, ok? I'm just sayin'..." – ☺ feeling happy

Jeanette

"You are fantastic, and I know that God will show up, show out, and guide you through a fantastic recovery, and you will use this trial as a testimony to bless others!"

Jim

"Dear Vivian, I'm sitting in a Bradley Center that's maybe 35% filled. Bucks are losing...again, and a certain, high-pitched voice is missing. Your team needs you, Viv. Get well soon."

Deidra

"Dear Vivian King. I was so happy to see you at the YWCA Racial Justice event on Tuesday. You are a true testament that God works miracles."

Valarie

"Hey, Viv! So glad to know that you are doing well! Hope to see you tonight at the appointed time and hour known to all *Scandal* addicts everywhere!"

Anique

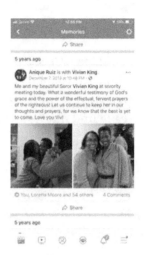

"Me and my beautiful Soror Vivian King at sorority meeting today. What a wonderful testimony of God's grace and the power of the effectual, fervent prayers of the righteous! Let us continue to keep her in our thoughts and prayers, for we know that the best is yet to come. Love you, Viv!"

Kimberla

"Vivian, I had no idea you'd been ill and just found out a couple of minutes ago. I am so happy to hear how well you're doing, and please know that I will certainly keep you in my prayers. Much love and God bless you always."

New to me was another social media platform called The Caring Bridge. Sona Mehring founded the website in 1997 after friends of hers had a premature baby and asked her to let everyone know. Instead of making dozens of emotional and time-consuming phone calls, she created the site that is used now for all types of health issues. June decided that this was the perfect way to alert those who had been expressing concerns about my health scare. Her first journal entry was on Halloween.

Journal entry by June Perry—Oct 31, 2013

Greetings friends . . . I know all of you are anxious to know what is happening with Vivian. She is progressing well and has a great appetite! Her bright smile has returned. But we are still asking that you do not visit the hospital. She needs a lot of uninterrupted rest and time to heal. Her mother is still here and is being taken care of by our Delta sisters and close friends.

I will keep you posted with any changes and let you know when she can go home, have visitors, etc.

This site also allows you to send Vivian a message!

There were fifteen comments in response to this first post. Here is just a sampling:

Kathy | *Nov. 1, 2013*

Vivian has been on my mind all week. Glad to know she is getting better. Miss her smile and funny Facebook posts. Praying for her complete healing. God bless.

Diane | *Nov. 2, 2013*

Love you, Vivian. Thinking about you every day, non-stop, and sending healing vibes out into the Universe for you!

Carrie | *Nov. 2, 2013*

Viv, know that *I love you* and that the good Lord is watching over you . . . Sam is wagging his tail extra fast right now, just for you!

> *"Sam is wagging his tail extra fast right now, just for you."*

Pat & Maurice | *Nov. 3, 2013*

Vivian, know that you are in our hearts and prayers. Take care to follow Doctor's orders, do everything that is expected of you to return to us full of life, spunk and joy that you bring to all around you. God is taking care of you in the manner that He always does . . . He loves you and will see you through this bump in your road.

Connie | Nov. 4, 2013

Vivian—I am so glad someone shared this with us. We are praying for you and are thrilled to hear you are recovering well. I'm sure you didn't have this planned in your busy schedule. We love you, and the girls said to tell Ms. Vivian to get well fast and I'm sure Bailey would too if she could talk. We are thinking about you!

Love, Craig and Connie

June's second journal entry was the next day, the one-week mark of my hospital stay.

Journal entry by June Perry— November 1, 2013

It is hard to believe that it has only been a week today since Vivian suffered a seizure while at the Girl Scouts breakfast at the Hyatt. The good thing is that she was surrounded by people who could get her medical attention right away. She could have been home alone, driving or not in a place where those who know and love her could make sure she got what she needed immediately. What a blessing!

She is progressing very well. The fact that she is very healthy mentally, physically and spiritually will speed this recovery process along. She is eating well and doing everything that the doctors, nurses and therapists ask of her. She also will express disdain at bad food :). So she ate two pieces of my pound cake (which she loves) at lunch and is having dinner delivered today by our good friend, Jennifer Bartolotta. *I am sure she will be very satisfied after this meal!*

I know you all want to talk to her, visit, etc. But send cards and well wishes. She still needs rest to allow her to recuperate. She may be moved from ICU to a regular room this evening or tomorrow but still no visitors...rest and recuperation is the prescription. Her Mom is going back to St. Louis tomorrow, but she will be back next week. We all know that this is a good sign because Mothers don't leave their children until they know things are going to be OK.

She knows you all love her, and she loves you all. I will keep you posted, and if there is something that I think any of you can do for her, I will certainly ask, and I know you will make it happen.

June Perry

This post received three times the response of the first message, with 46 comments. Here's just a sampling:

Johnna | Nov. 1, 2013

> *"Ummmm . . . I'm gonna need you to get better boo, ok!"*

Ummmm . . . I'm gonna need you to get better boo, ok! Thought about you again today (and every day) because the Bucks were playing the Celtics, and I thought to myself, me and Vivian would have been plotting on how to get to the game! Lol!

ReDonna | Nov. 2, 2013

The blessing of the Lord is here. I feel it in the atmosphere. The jubilant, vibrate, effervescent Viv will absorb all the love and prayers she is receiving as she heals. Her Mom feeling comfortable to go back to St. Louis definitely indicates she is getting stronger. Mothers don't leave nothing up to chance when it comes to their children. When Viv is well, the energy and love she is receiving will be magnified in the Community. Thank you, June, for keeping us updated. Thank you, everyone, for your prayers. We know how to love another.

Sara | Nov. 2, 2013

Vivian, my heart breaks for you. I'm sorry you are going through this difficult situation. I know you will recover and will grace us all with your eternal sunshine, smile, and amazing spirit very soon. Love you!

Barbara | Nov. 2, 2013

Hey, Vivian, Gurl, sending u lots of hugs and healing prayers. OK, I'll let u have Denzel for a day! lol Get well, Gurl. Gladiators from the heart! Hey, June.

Michele (Class of '83) | Nov. 2, 2013

Vivian, I am wishing you God speed and a full recovery very soon. My prayers will continue to be with you. God is in control, and I know he won't keep you down long. Stay faithful and positive, my sister. God bless you!!

Magda | Nov. 3, 2013

Vivian, you have had a huge spirit ever since 1st grade (and I'm sure well before that), and I feel certain that is going to pull you through. Lots of love from NYC.

Rose | Nov. 3, 2013

June—thank you for providing us an update on Vivian's progress. I'm glad to hear that her spirits are good, and she is progressing. Let us know if there is anything she needs. I was with her when this occurred and have been very concerned and agree relative to gratitude she was not alone.

Kelly | Nov. 4, 2013

Just seeing this news…hope you are feeling better. We are sending all kinds of love and good karma your way from Atlanta! XXOO

Four days later, June wrote the below entry, and a sampling of the twenty comments the post drew follows.

Journal entry by June Perry—Nov. 5, 2013

Greetings Vivian King Fan Club…Vivian is improving daily and has found things to laugh and be happy about! It is so good to see her smiling and enjoying the cards, notes and posts from you all. Her Mom is here, and Vivian's Delta Sorors have been taking very good care of her. Many of you have asked, "what can I do to help?" At this point, Vivian has everything she needs. Your thoughts and prayers are making all the difference in the world, so keep them coming! We will certainly let you know when she is ready for visitors.

June Perry

Jessica K. | Nov. 6, 2013

Vivian, I only heard today from Connie Jones about what happened to you. What a shocker! I was just wondering a couple of days ago what was making you so busy that you couldn't post on FB, cause that's not like you at all. Didn't expect this, of course. I'm very glad to read that you're improving, and I'll add my prayers to all the others for a fast recovery. Hope you quickly return to your bubbly self, the Vivacious Vivian King that we all know and love so much. And my thanks to June Perry for providing the updates.

XOXO

Jessica

Ryan | Nov. 7, 2013

Viv! So glad to hear of your progress! You are a trooper, so I know you'll be fine! Loving on you greatly from The Lou!! Sending you hugs and prayers! Sometimes GOD sits us down when we won't do it ourselves. I know this from experience. Be still and listen to what he is trying to tell you. Take time just to be in his presence and let him hold and comfort you. I love you, girl! Know and believe that!! Keep getting better!!

Anne E. | Nov. 7, 2013

Hey, Viv! Today on The Facebook (I know you love when I call it that), I asked your friends to post fav pix taken with you. I must love you because I posted the one of Mark and I with you and Raymond at the Black & White Ball, where my arm looks like a big ham hock! I love you and pray for you every day! I hope you like your impromptu photo album.

Hey, Viv! Today on The Facebook (I know you love when I call it that), I asked your friends to post fav pix taken with you.

Ron | *Nov. 7, 2013*

Vivian—it's great to hear that you are moving on the path toward recovery. Miss seeing you in the office and having the chance to talk about life, our work and the many interesting things that you seem to find time to do on your weekends. I live an exciting life through you . . . through the many trips and great experiences that you share through those conversations. I look forward to hearing more good news on your recovery and hope you are back on the 5th floor of the A building soon.

I was progressing well by June's November 8th post on The Caring Bridge.

Journal entry by June Perry — Nov. 8, 2013

Greetings to all of the Vivian King Fan Club Members! Just wanted you to know that Vivian is making great progress. Every day brings surprises at how she is able to persevere and do more than is expected of her! But that's Vivian, right? She is reading your posts here and on Facebook, so keep them coming! Cards and personal notes sent to St. Luke's Hospital, 2900 W. Oklahoma Ave. 53201 will get to her as well. Thanks for respecting her privacy and supporting her by allowing her to rest and recuperate.

There were twenty-four comments after this post. Here's a sampling.

Marlon | *Nov. 12, 2013*

Viv, Roz and I have you in deep rotation in our prayers. Give yourself whatever gifts of time and rest you need to feel better—and know that you're surrounded by caring thoughts and prayers and heartfelt wishes. Rest easy. Get well.

Kimberley | Nov. 13, 2013

Dear Lord, we thank you for your healing power. We thank you for the wonderful doctors, nurses and all the care providers who are supporting our sister's recovery. We thank you in advance for blessing Vivian with a return to health that enables her to continue being a light in the lives of so many. And we thank you for being omnipresent in Vivian's spirit so that she never forgets you are with her on this journey every step of the way and that You will bring her through. Those of us who adore her and miss her beautiful energy ask that you keep her encouraged, wrapping your loving spirit around her and being all that she needs. Thank you, God, for being there when we cannot, and thank you for hearing the prayers of every one of your Children petitioning on our Sister's

> *"Dear Lord, we thank you for your healing power."*

behalf, as we do what we can to show our love, support and faith in Vivian and importantly in You as you continue to bless Vivian. In Jesus' name, Amen.

Love, Portia | Nov. 15, 2013

Hello Vivian, I want you to know that I have been thinking of you and praying for your healing and recovery ever since I heard the news. You are a phenomenal woman, inside and out. May God give you and your family strength and ease any fears.

Dana | Nov. 16, 2013

Hey Viv. I'm happy to hear you're constantly improving. Ron, Jackson and I are always praying for you. Keep working hard.

As I was going through rehab, June slowed down on her posts. Her next one was on November 16. It was similar to the previous one. But there was good news on November 18. June saw the turning point that gave her confidence that I would make a full recovery.

Journal entry by June Perry — Nov. 18, 2013

Vivian is getting better and better every day! I am confident that she will be back to 100% soon. But don't stop the prayers, good wishes and positive thoughts. She still needs those.

Her caregivers are often amazed at what she can do, but we aren't surprised because we all know she is an overachiever! Her contagious smile is back, and she is anxious to get back on Facebook . . . and I bet it won't be long before she will be able to give you updates herself . . . so stay tuned!

June Perry

Patrice | Nov. 18, 2013

Fantastic to hear, but not surprising! =) Vivian, Pam Cullen said to tell you she's saying a prayer and to get well soon. I'm so glad you are on the mend! Don't wear yourself out overachieving!! Hugs.

> *"Don't wear yourself out overachieving!!"*

Andrew | Nov. 18, 2013

Hello Viv, I'm glad to hear that you're coming along. Keep up the good work. I spoke with your dad a while ago. Tell mom hello. Tell her that I can't get past the guards to see her (lol). You're in my prayers. My sister was here and sends her regards and well wishes to you. God bless you.

Melanie | Nov. 18, 2013

Hey Viv!!! Please know that you are in my thoughts and prayers!! I'm praying for a rapid recovery, but also that you will take this time to rest. God has a way of slowing us down when we need to. Trust in Him always! I am sure the hospital staff is enjoying having you as a temporary resident!! Lots of love to you!!

ReDonna | Nov. 18, 2013

When you have a healer that can touch every part of your being and a woman that is as faith-filled and spirited as our darling Viv, you know there is really going to be some healing. Love you, Vivian.

Ken | Nov. 19, 2013

Keep it going, Vivian. There's some Sushi out there missing you about now.

Carmen | Nov. 20, 2013

Thank you, June, for keeping us updated . . . I am happy to hear that you are getting better and better. I will continue to pray for you. I can't wait to hear what u have to say about *Scandal*! :) Miss and love you!

DeLinda | Nov. 22, 2013

Yay! Viv, I'm sooo happy to get this news. It is wonderful. Our house is cheering for you! I love you.

June's final post was very appropriate, considering my background.

Journal entry by June Perry — Nov. 22, 2013

Breaking news! Vivian has exceeded all expectations and will be released from the hospital early next week! Those special things that you all did for her . . . thoughts, prayers, food, flowers, etc. . . . made a huge difference in her ability to overcome obstacles and move forward with her life!

This is my last post on this site. I am sure Vivian will be in touch with you all . . . she can take it from here . . . and thanks so much!

June Perry

The sampling of the final responses matched June's enthusiasm:

Laura Cordell | Nov. 22, 2013

What an early Thanksgiving treat for You Vivian!!! June, I echo earlier comments. Thanks for keeping us posted so we could channel our positive thoughts and prayers Vivian's way!Top of Form

Riv | Nov. 24, 2013

June, thank you for caring so much for her and loving her and her friends enough to keep us posted and in the loop!! You are a jewel!! Can't thank you enough! Take care of yourself and Happy Holidays!!

Sadhna Lindvall | Nov. 26, 2013

HOORAY!!! We miss you!!!

As you can imagine, I was overwhelmed at the outpouring of support I received from social media. Thus, on December 5, 2013, I wrote this thank you on Facebook to the countless people, known and unknown, who prayed for me. June posted it on The Caring Bridge five days later.

> *"Thank you seems highly inadequate for everything that just happened to me, but it is all I have."*

Facebook Thank You:

My Dear Family, Sorors, Friends and Facebook Contacts,

Today is the day I was supposed to be released from the hospital. Instead, I left Aurora St. Luke's Medical Center nine days ago on November 26, two days before Thanksgiving. What would have been a 41-day stay turned into a 32-day stay, a remarkable recovery according to my doctor and therapists. I owe my progress thus far to all of them.

I know many of you are wondering what happened to me. It all began at an early morning breakfast. I arrived, greeted my table guests, and that is the last thing I completely remember until a couple of weeks later in the Neurological Intensive Care Unit at St. Luke's. From what I understand, I had a blood clot in my brain, which led to a stroke and then a seizure. Doctors cannot pinpoint exactly why it happened, but it had a profound impact on my body.

For 3 ½ weeks, I could not really talk, which I know would please some people. ☺ My right side lagged a bit. Physical Therapy has since brought that back to life. My speech is coming back nicely, but I still have outpatient therapy to go through until I am cleared to go back to work. I am not allowed to drive, so if anyone is going my way, give me a call. ☺

The first question one may ask during such a predicament is, 'why me?' Ironically, I never asked that question. I believe that is because I had a wonderful circle of care around me, determining what I needed, and unfortunately, that was not a lot of visitors. Here's where this becomes like the Academy Awards. Many of you have mentioned that my friend and soror, June Perry, was brilliant for keeping you updated on The Caring Bridge. I'd like to publicly thank June for setting that up to keep you abreast of my progress. I'd also like to thank June for helping many of my friends outside of Milwaukee accept what happened, coordinating extra food deliveries, and keeping me for a week during Thanksgiving so that my mother could go home.

I'd like to thank my friend and soror, Joan Prince, for being right there with June in limiting who was on the list to see me. She was also in charge of transportation, getting my mother to and from the hospital each evening and making sure she got food on certain days.

To Sorors Beverly Cooley, Jessica Murphy, Nuntiata Buck, and my good friend, Tracey Golden, thank you for your time and company during my recovery. Thank you for keeping people away so that I could concentrate on what I needed to do. Nuncie, Grant McLean and Darlene Jenkins Ray, thanks for feeding my mother. I thank Pastor John Wesley McVicker, Sr. and First Lady Marilynn McVicker for their prayers and visits and keeping Christ the King Baptist Church praying for me.

Thank you seems highly inadequate for everything that just happened to me, but it is all I have. I am overwhelmed by your cards, posts, flowers, gifts, but most of all, your prayers. I thank you from the bottom of my heart. Above all, I thank Almighty God for seeing me through this ordeal. He was with me each and every day, so to God be the Glory!

If you sent me something, rest assured that you WILL hear from me. It may take a little extra time, but I know that I want you to hear from me. It has been said that you never know who your friends are until you face a crisis. I have done that, and I am so pleased to call all of you my friends.

CHAPTER THIRTEEN

The Medicine

The big question is, why did I suffer from a stroke? What was the medical reason that led up to it? Nobody expected it. In fact, there was no obvious reason for anyone to expect it. From what my doctors told us, in addition to the research I have since done on strokes, I have pieced together the following explanation for what caused this interruption in my life.

Let's begin with the definition of a stroke. While many organizations have stroke information readily available on their websites, the Mayo Clinic has one of the most comprehensive pages I've seen. It says a stroke occurs when the blood supply to parts of your brain is interrupted or reduced, depriving brain tissue of oxygen and nutrients. It also breaks down strokes a little further. There are three kinds of strokes: ischemic, hemorrhagic, and transient ischemic attack or TIA, which is a temporary disruption of blood flow to the brain. About 80% of strokes are ischemic, and I was in that 80% of patients.

The medical field gets even more specific by defining the two types of ischemic strokes: thrombotic and embolic. A thrombotic stroke occurs when a blood clot or thrombus forms in one of the arteries that supply blood to your brain. An embolic stroke occurs when a blood clot or other debris forms away from your brain and is swept through your bloodstream to lodge in narrower brain arteries. I had a thrombotic stroke.

However, doctors said my stroke was even rarer because it was not the usual arterial type. One of the physicians on my case wrote a book for practitioners called, "FAST: Stroke Guide." Dr. Akram Shhadeh said my stroke was a venous stroke or in the veins leading into my heart. This cerebral venous thrombosis (CVT) caused blood stasis or stagnation and caused pressure within my veins to increase to the point that the veins leaked into my brain tissue and caused bleeding.

The Mayo Clinic also says a stroke can cause a seizure, a sudden, uncontrolled electrical disturbance in the brain. A seizure is exactly what alerted the people around me at the Girl Scouts Breakfast on October 25, 2013. I would have a second one before I left the premises. So, on that fateful day, a blood clot formed on the left side of my brain over the part of the brain that manages speech. At some point, this clot in my veins caused pressure, and my veins started leaking, causing intracranial bleeding, or bleeding within my skull. The bleeding killed brain cells, which led to my aphasia or inability to speak.

Some of the notes listed in my health records were the following:

- Venous sinus thrombosis

- Intracranial hemorrhage

- Seizure

To monitor what was happening with my brain, I was subjected to several Magnetic Resonance Imaging (MRI) scans. MRIs use powerful magnets, radio waves and a computer to take detailed pictures inside your body. Doctors use MRIs to diagnose a disease or injury. They also help monitor how well a patient is responding to treatment. The MRIs I underwent did both of those for me. To minimize my chance of having another seizure, I was given Keppra*, which is the brand name of levetiracetam. I was also prescribed that for another year after I left the hospital.

To keep my blood thin to reduce clotting, I was given the anticoagulant Warfarin or Coumadin. I had to keep that up after I left the hospital, as well, with some dietary considerations. Managing my anticoagulation therapy meant a weekly trip to the Anti-Coagulation Clinic at St. Luke's, and it was tricky because you have to pay attention to the vitamin K you ingest.

At each appointment, I would have what's called a PT-INR test. This stands for Prothrombin Time-International Normalized Ratio. The ClotCare Online Resource has a wealth of knowledge about anticoagulation therapy, but basically, the PT portion of the test measures how quickly your blood clots. The INR is the standard unit used to report the result of a PT test. ClotCare states that "the most common INR target range for someone on Warfarin is somewhere between 2.0 and 4.0." My target was 3.0 – 3.5. INRs of 5.0 or more are to be avoided. If your blood is 5.0 or more, you are basically in danger of bleeding to death.

Those television commercials about blood thinners may have a pleasant voice delivering the news that this product "may cause fatal bleeding," but it is, unfortunately, the truth. I decided to wear only flat shoes at this time—very uncharacteristic of me—because I did not want to fall on the winter ice or uneven payment and bleed to death. I would joke about it with my friends. They did not particularly like those jokes. I suppose it was the humor that helped me deal with this potential.

Anyway, when you have these PT-INR tests, the nurse who administers it gives you a list of instructions with all the factors that can adversely impact your weekly readings. You have to report any changes in habits—medicine, nutritional supplements, exercise regimen, alcohol use or diet—to your clinician each week, especially if you are outside of your target INR window. This is where we talked about vitamin K. The issue is that vitamin K plays a vital role in the body's natural clotting process. Here's how ClotCare explains it:

> *"Your liver uses vitamin K to make blood-clotting proteins. Warfarin works against vitamin K. Warfarin reduces your liver's ability to use vitamin K to produce normally functioning forms of the blood clotting proteins. Therefore, warfarin reduces your risk of forming a blood clot."*

The bottom line is that any change in your vitamin K intake can make your INR rate fluctuate. You don't have to stay away from vitamin K. You just need to be consistent with your intake, and that's hard when all of your favorite vegetables have high vitamin K content: broccoli, spinach, Bibb, and red leaf lettuce, cabbage, Brussels sprouts, and all of the greens my grandmother used to make. Yes, collard, mustard *and* turnips. A foodie like me can easily forget the vitamin K intake, or worse, overdo. Still, I tried to log all of my food so that I could have an accurate report for my clinician each week.

Alcohol can definitely thin your blood out. While I was told I could have an occasional glass of wine, I got "caught up" as they say, when I went to an out-of-town conference in March. We were talking and having a good time after a long day of workshops. It was just one night. I did not think anything of it until my next appointment recorded my INR as 5.2. Yikes!

"Maybe I need to bar you from going out of town," my clinician said at my next appointment.

I promised her that it would not happen again. Doctors also used medicine while I was in Neurological Intensive Care to keep my brain from swelling. A neurosurgeon was on stand-by, just in case my brain swelled to the point of needing surgery. Fortunately, doctors did not have to take such measures.

"During the beginning stages, your poor mom would grab your hand, and she would rub it," said Jessica. "She'd say, 'Say my name, Vivian. What is my name? Vivian, what is my name?' And you would just look at her, and you would smile, and she'd say, 'Come on, Vivian, you know my name.' "

Then Jessica would try to help, as the doctors had asked my care circle to do. "I would write down on paper, 'Mom,'" Jessica said. "And you would go, 'Mom.'"

This would encourage my mother.

"She'd say, 'Yes, I am Mom, but what is my name?'" Jessica said. "And she was just rubbing your hands and begging you to talk. And at that point, you couldn't get the words out."

The Centers for Disease Control says on its website that African American women are twice as likely to have a stroke as white women. They also are more likely to have strokes at younger ages and to have more severe strokes. So, as we searched for answers as to what caused my stroke, being an African American woman was one factor.

Back to the Mayo Clinic, its stroke information page outlines other common risk factors. It lists the following lifestyle risk factors:

- Being overweight or obese

- Physical inactivity

- Heavy or binge drinking

- Use of illicit drugs, such as cocaine or methamphetamines

According to my Body Mass Index (BMI) at the time, I was in the low area of the overweight category. You're overweight if you have a BMI between 25 and 29.9, and mine was 26.6 at the time. However, I was pretty active in my job and in the gym or walking outside occasionally. Plus, I am a social drinker, not a heavy one, and I do not use illicit drugs. The Mayo Clinic goes on to list medical risk factors:

- Blood pressure readings higher than 120/80 millimeters of mercury (mm Hg)

- Cigarette smoking or exposure to secondhand smoke

- High cholesterol

- Diabetes

- Obstructive sleep apnea

- Cardiovascular disease, including heart failure, heart defects, heart infection or abnormal heart rhythm

- Personal or family history of stroke, heart attack or transient ischemic attack

I did not and still do not have high blood pressure and do not smoke. (I tried smoking as a teenager and decided it was not for me.) I did not have high cholesterol or diabetes. I had not been diagnosed with sleep apnea or any cardiovascular disease. Additionally, I do not have a history of stroke or heart attack in my family, although my uncle passed unexpectedly in 2018 of a heart attack at the age of 71.

Finally, the Mayo Clinic clearly lists other factors associated with a higher risk of stroke, and that's where my risks show up.

- Age—People 55 or older have a higher risk of stroke than do younger people

- Race—African Americans have a higher risk of stroke than do people of other races

- Sex—Men have a higher risk of stroke than women.

- Hormones—use of birth control pills or hormone therapies that include estrogen, as well as increased estrogen levels from pregnancy and childbirth

At 49, I was still considered relatively young to have a stroke. Again, being African American is a factor. Here is where the birth control shows up. I had been taking birth control pills for a few years, at this point, because I decided to be sexually active again. My OB/GYN at the time did not seem to have a problem with it, so there I was, over forty and taking birth control pills. For some reason, estrogen or hormone therapy increases a woman's chance of developing blood clots. I have also read that stress or anxiety slows down blood flow and can cause clotting. The doctors shared this information with my care circle.

"They had realized that the only medicine you were on was the birth control," Nuncie told me. 'That's when [the doctor] said the imbalance of the medicine that does the hormone balance was the longevity of it, taking it for so long. He said it's on there, every side effect, but it's not something people really think about. It was the imbalance that caused the clot and the clot that caused the stroke."

This news triggered a discussion about the man in my life at the time. June, apparently, picked up her phone, stating that they should let Raymond and my mother know this latest information. Nuncie launched back into protection mode.

"Time out. You don't need to let Raymond know nothing right now," Nuncie said. "That may be right now Vivian's love of her life, but he is not the end-all-be-all, and he does not need to know anything about the fact of her personal life and what she's been doing. Vivian may not want him to know that she's been on birth control. It ain't his business. It ain't nobody's business right now."

"Yeah, Nuncie, I kind of agree with you," said Joan. "I don't think we need to share that right now."

Out of the complications the Mayo Clinic lists for strokes, I had three of the six.

- Paralysis or loss of muscle movement

- Difficulty talking or swallowing

- Memory loss or thinking difficulties

I did not have identified emotional problems, pain or changes in behavior and self-care ability.

There is good news on the Mayo Clinic website and about strokes these days. They can be treated and prevented. In fact, the CDC estimates up to 80% of strokes can be prevented. Most importantly, though, many fewer Americans die of stroke now than in the past. I am most fortunate to fall into these statistics. There is no doubt in my mind that if I had stayed at home on the morning of October 25, 2013, I would not be here to write this book.

PART III

The Lessons

CHAPTER FOURTEEN

What's Really on Your Mind?

Tracey Golden is my unofficial therapist. If I paid her, she would make a fortune, but she's content with being my close friend, my sister in Christ, if you will, gently guiding my mental wellness with every one of our conversations. I mentioned before how we originally met at church, and she was on my list of "sisters" allowed to visit me in the hospital when I landed in Neurological ICU. What I failed to mention is that she earned her master's degree in Community Psychology from Alverno College and now has her own counseling business.

It's interesting that Tracey came to visit me quite often at the hospital, yet she seemed to miss the crowds. That's really how she prefers it, though. People are drawn to her because of her amazing presence and welcoming and non-judgmental personality, but she can do without a lot of people around, even though she quietly commands attention in a crowd.

We sat down in her meticulously clean but comfortable kitchen to talk about her take on my stroke and that entire period in our lives. Her dog, Jackson, the cutest little blonde Bichon- Poodle mix you ever will meet, had finally tired of jumping up to lick me and get the over-the-top attention I normally give him. Tracey remembered being in her back cottage, preparing to leave for work, when June called her on October 25.

"She was very calm, which made me feel very calm," begins Tracey. "It was clear to me that she was trying to ensure that I would be calm. Then she told me about it, and she told me you were OK and that you were at the hospital."

Tracey can't remember if she went straight to the hospital when she heard, but she knows that she did make it to St. Luke's that day. I was sleeping when she arrived.

"When you did open your eyes, it seemed clear to me that you recognized me," said Tracey. "But it was as if something wasn't connecting. You weren't speaking."

Tracey actually visited me multiple times during my hospital stay. From the beginning, she says she knew I was going to be fine. When I asked her about why she had this perspective, this is when my interview with her somehow turned into one of those impromptu therapy sessions.

"Because you were still here," Tracey said. "I mean, it's one of those things. Maybe you weren't sure that you wanted to stay, which may have contributed to the actual stroke on a spiritual level, but you were still here, and you wouldn't want to be here any other way. So, it was just one of those things where 'she will be fine.' So, I just pictured you as being fine."

Tracey believes I recognized her every time she came to visit. She said I never looked scared or seemed to question with my eyes, 'who is this strange person coming into my room?' It also seemed to be really quiet when Tracey visited, so often, she would just sit in the corner and pray and know that I was going to be OK.

"I remember a time when I was sitting in the room with you, and they brought you food, and you couldn't navigate the silverware. I think it may have been soup," Tracey said. "I unwrapped stuff for you, and you looked at the silverware and picked up the knife, and it was as if you thought, 'no, that's not right. That's not gonna work.' I kinda just let you work with it for a little while, and I just came over to the bed 'cause I was thinking, 'she's not ready for that part yet.' So, I just fed you whatever it was that they brought, and you smiled."

Tracey and I then talked a little about my risk factors, which were minimal. This information bears repeating: I did not have high blood pressure. I do not have a history of stroke in my family, and I was relatively young compared to the average stroke victim. Doctors pointed to birth control pills over the age of forty as the primary factor, in addition to my being African American. Essentially, a white woman with a similar lifestyle and credentials is two times less likely to have a stroke. Tracey understood the risk of birth control pills but shared her story.

"I've been taking birth control pills over forty for ten years," said Tracey. "And I think that does play a role. I also think that things that are happening with us emotionally and the unspoken stuff—I'll just call it spiritual stuff—has a huge role."

I was looking at Tracey deeply at this point and pondering her words as she talked.

"It's having experience with lack of ease, which is why there's dis-ease," Tracey said. "Something's happening, and maybe you don't realize something is happening because it doesn't look different from anybody else you know or it feels like this is what's supposed to be. But when illness comes, when there *is* dis-ease, there's a spiritual component to it, a psychological component to it, and I don't know that we always look at the way we're thinking about things."

Now Tracey really had me thinking, particularly thinking back to what was going on at the time of my stroke.

"It doesn't have to be an illness. It can be the way we think about how our lives have unfolded or *are* unfolding," Tracey said. "It can be what we think about what we want as opposed to what we've got. It can be about how close am I to the things that I want? Do I believe I can have what I want? A lot of the time, the discrepancy between what I want and what I believe I can have can cause a great deal of illness. Because we're here in this physical body to be, do, have whatever we want, and when we think we can't have it, that's a problem, and it manifests itself in physical ways."

Finally, this thought process ended for her, and I was listing in my mind what was manifesting itself in my life in the fall of 2013. After all, I was three months into an exciting new job. It was a promotion to a Vice President from my previous Director role at a different company. It was quite a challenge because I was charged with building a new department to serve in the area of Community Relations. I was in a relationship and having a fun year with my love. I was about to travel to Texas to see an NFL football game in the new Dallas Cowboys' stadium. I felt like I was "on cloud nine," a common expression to demonstrate one's height of happiness.

"That's the thing. You're so non-stop," said Tracey. "I don't know that you always are knowing, attentive to what's happening."

I sort of pouted at this statement, as I thought that I was self-aware.

"You are, usually, on cloud nine," she said. "But there are some things that go through your mind that you just tell to keep moving, that could probably use a little bit of love and attention in order to just get you into alignment with who you are. Does that make sense at all?"

While I did not want it to, it was making perfectly good sense. It was at that point that I realized, I should go back and examine any journals that I kept around the time of my stroke to understand what was really on my mind at the time.

Tracey interrupted my thoughts.

"It was interesting. I ran into Brad at the grocery store," she said.

Brad Pruitt is an award-winning filmmaker from Milwaukee whose series on gun violence has been used as a tool by schools, universities, community organizations, and prisons to help examine the critical issue of gun violence. As a filmmaker, he is always observing his surroundings and trying to determine their impact on people. I had seen him at an event a few weeks before and shared with him the topic of this book.

"A point that he brought up, which is something that he probably said to you, was about how he started to notice that women in his life, black women, around the same age, were coming up with these medical conditions or having these medical events," said Tracey. "And he said, he really thought, *what in the world is going on? What is this?* And he started to look at the commonalities between them."

The common qualities he noticed:

- Women who are doing really well

- Corporate women, for the most part

- High-powered, high-pressure careers

- Often single

"And he said it doesn't make sense," said Tracey. "What I said to him in response to that was, 'a lot of times, people can think that the stress that they're feeling with work is normal.'"

One of the women Brad used as an example was told that her natural hair was not appropriate for work.

"There are so many ways that people can beat you up or suggest that you're not all that you need to be, and that can have an impact, even if you don't realize it's having an impact," Tracey said. "Oftentimes, what we do is group together, and we say, 'They're on some bullshit.' Yeah, they are, and we conform, and we keep moving, and we don't really address what's happening inside of us because of that statement."

In such an instance, Tracey said we don't stop and ask how that impacted us or even examine if it did impact us. We don't ask what's going on with us. We just know that we're OK and we keep moving.

Our self-talk is, "We're so strong. It's happening to everybody. It's not a big deal, and we discount it."

"If someone stabs you in the arm every morning, it becomes a non-event, but it is having an impact on your body," said Tracey. "At some point, your arm's not gonna work the same."

"And psychologically, something's not gonna work the same," she continues. "So, it can be a lot of little, I've heard them called microaggressions, in the workplace. A lot of little things that in and of themselves may not seem to be significant, but when you look at them over a twenty to thirty-year career, or you look at them over a group, a culture, especially within the dynamic of race, you can come up with some stuff that can be pretty traumatizing that remains unaddressed."

Tracey's words were a lot for me to unpack. They had me thinking about the fact that I let a lot of things roll off my back because I always feel that somebody has it worse than I do, so why should I complain? At the very least, why should I make a big deal out of it?

"It's interesting to me that you didn't have a timeline, but you had these things that you wanted to do," Tracey said. Then she shares one story about her work.

"I have a client who's in her mid-thirties, corporate woman. She's not black, and she came to see me because her timeline hadn't been met, and she was saying there's anxiety around that. Now a black woman's never going to talk to someone about 'I'm here, and this isn't where I planned to be,'" said Tracey.

"This woman wasn't distraught," Tracey said. "But she felt it, and because she felt it, she was like, 'I'm gonna go talk to somebody about this.'"

Then Tracey said something that really rang true for me, as I think about my life and the lives of many of my like-minded friends.

"The world could come to an end, and we'd be like, 'I got this. I got this. I don't need to talk to anybody. Everybody else is going through the same shit I'm going through. I got this. It ain't nothing. I got this,'" she said theatrically. "I think it's manifesting in people. Brad was separating it out, making distinctions, but I don't really see differences."

I laughed at her comment. Seriously, though, from a faith perspective, I would probably be asking, "What does God want me to learn from this?" And I know a lot of my Christian friends would be asking the same thing. We'd probably get a glass of wine, as Tracey and I were drinking at that moment, and turn on a *Law & Order* rerun convinced it would all be OK in the morning.

"Culturally, I think for African-American women, we have gotten so accustomed to not feeling good that that's the norm," Tracey interrupted my thoughts again.

"And not that you don't feel good, but when something happens that doesn't feel good, or I don't even know if most of us notice that we're feeling depressed, depression or any of these things because we don't seem to expect to be way up here," Tracey stated as she held one hand above her head. "It's just that whatever happens, I can handle."

"Probably more like whatever happens I *have* to handle," I interjected.

"Yes, yes," Tracey said. "So getting help is not an option. Jackson!"

Tracey sternly calls her dog's name because while we were talking, he had gotten hold of the toilet paper from the nearby bathroom and had strewn it all on the floor under the table where we were sitting. Once Tracey cleaned up after Jackson and sat back down, she started talking about the time leading up to my stroke.

"I think I hadn't seen you very much," she said. "I remember thinking, 'What's going on with her? What's happening in your life that would contribute to this?'"

We started talking again about what doctors say likely caused my stroke, birth control pills over the age of forty. Tracey's curious that my OB/GYN wouldn't have pointed out my age and asked if I still wanted to take them. I was more curious about why she was still taking them.

"Well, I guess that I figure it is what it is," she said. "I have to take them, or my body just kinda goes berserk. So, I'm on the lowest possible dosage."

When I asked what she meant by berserk, she continued explaining.

"If I don't have them, I'll get sick every month, violently ill, lose twenty pounds, throw up for two days. It is insane," she said, with a pained look on her face at the thought of it. As the image of her on the floor hanging over the toilet, violently ill crossed my mind, I was glad that I did not have such menstrual cycles.

We were finally at the last question that I had asked each of my interview subjects. Looking at me today, knowing what you witnessed, what are your thoughts?

"This is what I expected you to be," Tracey said. "In my mind, I told myself that the most important thing that I could do to help you was to picture you well. And so, I couldn't see you any other way because I thought that's of no service to her. So that's what I had to do."

So, Tracey pictured me well. And I got well, despite my thirty-two-day hospital stay. Tracey chuckled at her next thought, imagining my posture when I decided to go ahead and throw a fiftieth birthday party for myself nearly a year later. I had originally planned a trip to South Africa in August, which I took. However, when I returned and my birthday was coming up in October, I thought, *how am I going to celebrate on my actual birthday?* That's when my African-themed party idea was born.

"Like with your birthday," Tracey said as she began telling the story of what I would say if someone asked why they weren't invited. "You were like, 'You know I had a neurological event. That's why you didn't make the list.' And I was thinking, *'Yep, I knew this would happen.'* When you started leveraging, I thought, *'Yep, mmm hmm. That's my girl right there.'"*

Tracey's husband walked in from work and changed clothes to take Jackson for his afternoon walk. Tracey was relieved so that she didn't have to worry about any more tissue incidents.

"I know that you have friends who 'know you know you,'" Tracey said. "But people on the outside looking in, those who want to have a piece of you to do this or ask if you can come to that, they don't 'know you know you.'"

She paused and then continued.

"You at the core of your being are just loving, easy-going, let God have His way," she said.

I am listening intently again and thinking, *true.*

"But when you start piling on what people think about you and what you've done, and how they perceive your accomplishments, and how they perceive you and the value that they perceive that they can get from doing this with you or that with you, and all these other things," she said. "And then with you at your core being loving, easy-going, fun, if they present something and a reason why you should do it, a lot of times, you're *in.*"

We both burst out laughing at the sheer truth of what she was saying.

"Get *out!*" Tracey said. "Stop being *in* all the time. OK, I can do that. I can do that. That sounds like fun. And then you get them excited about it, which is great, but you cannot go 24/7."

I am speechless at this discourse at this point.

"There's so much pulling on you," Tracey said. "You thrive, and you make it all happen. It's not like balls are dropping."

"Except for my house," I said.

I finally spoke up again with an image of my messy bedroom and closet in my head.

"But you're exhausted. You're exhausted," Tracey said. "And your house, and all these things that would really nurture you, you're letting go because of this demand and that demand and I gotta do this because this is expected and that's expected, and you're all over the place all of the time."

"I hadn't thought of it like that," I said.

"I think that Brad makes a very valid point about how culturally, groups of people, like black women in America who are single, or I don't know, whomever," Tracey said. "You can definitely look at groups of people and find commonalities. Like this is how we navigate these things."

Tracey pauses in thought and then continues speaking.

"Or like black women saying I have to make it through and just persevering no matter what and not necessarily tending to themselves."

She then turns her words directly to my particular situation.

"But I think more than anything, it's not necessarily a culture that's pressing on you like that. I think it's just that 'I'm Vivian. I have more energy than one person ought, and I'm going to spend it, all of it. Today. Everyday. I'm spending everything, spending it all. Living my best life every day, all day, nonstop. I might not even drink too much water, so I don't have to miss too much by going to the bathroom. You are that . . .'"

Tracey ended her sentence with a gesture symbolizing something just going, going and going, like the Energizer Bunny from the battery commercials.

I was literally silent. Not saying anything, just thinking about everything Tracey just said, when she asked me a question.

"Do you remember when you finally got home, and you were doing things, and I was like, two things a day?"

I nodded my head in the affirmative.

"You got out [of the hospital] wanting to do this and this and this," Tracey said. "And I was like Vivian, two things, just two things."

Now I was thinking about years ago when Tracey made this point to me.

"I remember you telling me, 'You do more things in a weekend than most people have done in a year,'" I said.

"You *do*," Tracey said.

Again, we both laughed.

"I guess I just don't like missing experiences because experiences are rich," I said, trying to explain.

At the time of our conversation, we were about a week past the United Negro College Fund Gala. I started telling Tracey about how I had missed it and actually forgot that it was coming up. In my old job, I would have had it on the calendar and filled our company table. On my sabbatical at this time, I felt like I wasn't in the loop anymore. I told Tracey that I almost "got in my feelings," and then I stopped and said to myself, "Vivian, you can't make every party."

"I'm glad you're out of the loop," Tracey said. "'Cause that loop was killing you."

We laughed as the back door opened in the background.

Jackson came bursting into the house from his walk and greeted me like he normally did, jumping and licking. This therapy session was officially over.

CHAPTER FIFTEEN

What I've Learned

Before I landed at St. Luke's for more than a month, I had only been in the hospital as a patient when I underwent surgery to remove fibroids in my uterus. Other than that, I had always only *visited* others in the hospital. At the time of my stroke, I was a new Vice President of Community Relations at Aurora Health Care with communications and community relations experience but no real experience in health care. My health ordeal changed all of that. I became a first-hand witness to the care we delivered in our health care system.

I now knew how nurses went about their day, checking on patients and making sure we were comfortable. I now knew the necessity of occupational therapy, how physical therapy really does make you stronger, and how speech therapy helps you not only relearn how to say words but how to write them. I learned that you need an advocate with you during your serious medical appointments, especially if you are incapacitated in some way. I learned that faith is not just reserved for the patient, but caregivers often have faith, as well.

I have come to learn that strokes are like fingerprints. Each one is different, and each one has its own impact on your life. This stroke taught me the importance of what I now call "the three Ps." When faced with a health situation or any major challenge in life, you need a posse, persistence, and prayer.

My posse launched into action right away, knowing that I was the only person in my family living in Wisconsin. Fortunately, there were people around me during my health scare who knew I had a posse, and the calls began going out. The news spread like wildfire or went viral, depending on your era.

"We were fast and furious between texts and emails, sending information to people," said Nuncie.

While my posse had a few extra people in it, it was mostly made up of members of my sorority, Delta Sigma Theta. I have always felt that Delta women are powerful, but this ordeal showed me the true power of our sisterhood. It reminded me of the rings that are formed when you throw a pebble into a pond. The action causes a wave of rings that gradually gets wider. My inner ring was at the hospital, but they reached out to other sorors, and *they* reached out to even more.

"I did call the State Chaplain and let her know that you were in the hospital," said Jessica. "And I said, 'Peggy, can you please pray for my sister?'"

"What happened?" Peggy asked.

"And I told her, and then when I came back up [to the hospital] that night, she and Soror Gaines had come and prayed with you and put oil on you," said Jessica.

In the hierarchy of Delta Sigma Theta, you have your national leadership, your regional leadership, and then the state leadership that serves as direct liaisons to individual chapters. Rev. Peggy, an ordained minister, was our State Chaplain, and Carola Gaines was the president of the Madison Alumnae Chapter. They both lived in Madison, Wisconsin, and drove the hour and fifteen minutes to Milwaukee after Jessica's call. Jessica was our State Coordinator at the time.

"That really touched our spirit that they came all the way from Madison to do that," said Jessica. "I remember it like yesterday when I got that call."

My TV sisterhood was also a major part of my posse. Susan drove us to a therapy appointment one day, Kim's husband, Rick, and Katrina dropped off food at my place.

"I got all those healthy foods from my healthy trainer person," said Kim. "For some reason, I couldn't deliver it, so I made Rick deliver it. And you were cracking me up because you said you thought it was some random delivery person named Rick when he called from the lobby."

Not too long after Rick's delivery, Katrina came over with more food.

Katrina said, "I remember going to the grocery store and getting all of your staples, like milk and eggs, and some of your personal list of favorites. At least you guys were getting set up where your mom didn't have to leave. That was the biggest thing. Nobody had to leave the house to take care of anything."

When I asked the girls why they did all of this, their answers were simple and profound.

" 'Cause we love you," said Susan.

"We do. We love you," said Katrina. "And you would've done the exact same thing for us."

"And on top of all the emotional love, we're all doers," said Kim. "We wanted to make sure you were taken care of in terms of coming home and recovering and not having to worry about food. That's what we do - just make things happen."

"Kimmy was executive-producing your arrival home," said Susan.

That made us all laugh. You never really know how you impact people. I did not realize how many people genuinely cared for me and did not want me to leave this earth just yet.

You have read about most of them throughout this book, but two people who formerly lived in Milwaukee felt helpless in their new cities.

James Lynch lived in Seattle. He was outside of his apartment, leaning into his girlfriend's car, telling her I had had a stroke. "Not hearing Vivian's voice . . .," James said. "I was happy when you started talking again."

Crystal McNeal had moved to Nashville, her first job outside of Milwaukee. "I felt so badly that I was far away. I couldn't be there. I couldn't visit. I just immediately prayed. Lord, she's gotta get through this. It's not her time."

Having worked with James at two television stations during my career and with Crystal through mutual journalism and public relations organizations in Milwaukee, they will tell you that I am persistent in reaching my goals once I set them and put my mind to it. Throughout my life, I have been that way. I was often the teacher's pet in school, if you will. When I set out to get jobs, I would get this feeling of sheer confidence when I really wanted and adequately prepared for a job, to the point of knowing that it was mine if I wanted it.

For example, when I interviewed for my second TV job in Tyler, Texas, they told me I was a finalist but that they ended up offering it to a woman in San Antonio. My spirit was so confused, as I really thought that was my next job. I almost started to doubt myself. Two days later, the assistant news director called me to tell me they wanted to offer me the job after all. The other candidate's station counter-offered to keep her, and I was next in line. I *knew* that was my job.

I share that story to illustrate my persistence when I put my mind to it. It was the same persistence I needed to restore me to wellness after my stroke. At the beginning of my hospital stay, I was clueless as to why I was there. I did not fully comprehend that I had suffered a stroke, and I did not even remember that I was a broadcaster. Once I was in therapy and knew that I should already know some of the things they were trying to teach me, I felt inadequate. But I became the teacher's pet again. I set my mind to achieving or exceeding at all the tasks each therapist put in front of me.

In my quiet time, I also began to reflect on my relationship with Raymond. I wanted to see him so badly, but he remained in Los Angeles. During one of my conversations with him, I shared that I wished he had come to visit. That's when he told me that he felt helpless when June called him about my stroke, and his first inclination was to try to figure out how he was going to get to Milwaukee. Once he got to Milwaukee, he planned to stay at my place. Then he shared with me a conversation he had with my mother after June told him he needed to talk to Mom.

"She said to me, 'Can you afford to come to Milwaukee? And if you come, you will have to stay at a hotel because I am staying at Vivian's, and I don't think her sorors are prepared to take you back and forth like they are doing for me,' " Raymond said. "I was having financial problems. I couldn't afford a hotel."

I was flabbergasted at this story. I confirmed this with my mother later, and she shared the same details, almost verbatim.

"I remember talking to my mom about this, and I asked her if I should go anyway," Raymond said. "And she said, 'Naw, don't go.' In hindsight, I should've put my foot down with your mom. I honestly say I wasn't there for you as much as I should've been. I do regret that."

I live with few regrets. I really think things happen for a reason, and I think this was God's way of helping me figure out that Raymond and I should not be together after all. I joked with my friends at the time, telling them that my mother was a gangster and "punked" Raymond. I guess that was my way of using a little humor to cope with losing a love. No matter how you describe it, I felt that if Raymond could not be there for me when I was near death, what would happen when other challenges arose in our lives? We broke up in January, shortly after I went back to work. I wanted to be persistent in getting to the life God had planned for me.

Finally, as a Christian, this experience reminded me that God is in control, "And we know that all things work together for good to them that love God, to them who are the called according to his purpose" (Romans 8:28). As I reflect on that scripture, I realize that God was with me from the very beginning. The dictionary defines "coincidence" as "a striking occurrence of two or more events at one time apparently by mere chance." To me, God and coincidence are interchangeable. So, here is how I knew God was with me throughout my experience.

- I woke up on October 25, not feeling like going to the Girl Scouts breakfast. I decided to go anyway, which put me in a public place where I could receive immediate attention.

- I worked for the largest health care system in the state, so my employer knew I was not just calling in sick. My CEO was kept abreast of the seriousness of my situation, and not only did he send a handwritten note expressing his concern and wishing me a speedy recovery, but he shared with my care team that I should not worry about what would happen to my new job in my absence. It would be there when I returned.

- Though I had only been at my job just under four months when I suffered my stroke, I had sketched out a plan for my department based on my impressions of the first ninety days. When I returned to work part-time in January, the company had restructured. If I had begun my work, I would've had to re-introduce my plan to leaders. So, while it was not my first choice to have a stroke, God's timing made everything OK.

- God blessed the relationships I have so much that I had a firm posse in place. He also blessed my mother in the same way. My posse was taking care of us in Milwaukee with food and all of our needs, while her posse held things down with my father and grandmother in St. Louis, taking care of all of their needs.

- The Bible encourages you to "pray continually." In fact, the King James Version of 1 Thessalonians 5:17 reads, "Pray without ceasing." I had a lot of prayers being said for me all over the world.

Thanks to all of the above, I no longer have a spirit of worry. My motto when I got out of the hospital was "Don't sweat the small stuff," because 99.9% of the things we generally worry about are so small in the whole scheme of things. Instead of worrying, we need to seek God in all things, and He will provide you with a peace that surpasses all understanding.

Lamentations 3:25 states, "The Lord is good to those whose hope is in Him, to the one who seeks Him."

Philippians 4: 6–7 in the New International Version states, "Do not be anxious about anything, but in every situation, by prayer and petition, with thanksgiving, present your requests to God. And the peace of God, which transcends all understanding, will guard your hearts and your minds in Christ Jesus."

I ultimately learned that prayer is needed for all challenges. God expects prayer for all things. And we all learned that God still performs miracles. I am a living example.

CHAPTER SIXTEEN

Telling My Story

What I know for sure is that my story can help someone. I ultimately realized this when I first shared my testimony in public. On New Year's Eve 2013, I attended Christ the King Baptist Church's New Year's Eve service. Like many African American churches, my congregation holds what's called a watch night service at 10 p.m. on December 31. Sometimes we do it by ourselves; other times, we may share the service with another congregation. Their members either come to our church or vice versa.

The history of watch night services dates back to the Civil War and slavery in America. Many free and freed blacks living in the Union States, and slaves on plantations, were said to have gathered in churches and other safe spaces on New Year's Eve in 1862 to await word that the Emancipation Proclamation had been signed into law by President Abraham Lincoln on January 1, 1863. Back then, the enslaved and freed stood, knelt and prayed while they waited. Modern-day services provide singing, praying and preaching but also an opportunity for congregations to review the past year and pray about doing better in the year ahead.

Testimonies are most important during watch night services because time is specifically set aside for them. People are passionate when they give them, and there are typically several given during the service. For years, I listened to testimonies of people who overcame an alcohol or drug addiction, domestic violence or financial difficulties. Other people had come through health issues, lost a job and rebounded, or thanked God for family resolutions. I listened, always thinking that I never had such serious situations, so I was reluctant to get up to share my first-world problems, if you will. After my stroke, I finally felt that what I had to say was worth getting up and walking to the microphone.

I remember standing in a short line until it was my turn. I also remember being a little nervous. Sure, I had spoken in front of a crowd before—and certainly in front of the television camera's eye with tens of thousands of viewers behind it—but I had never up to this point offered a personal testimony in this way. I began telling my story, that on October 25th of that year, I had awakened feeling fine. My only thought was that I really did not want to get up and go to the breakfast I had been invited to, but I decided to go anyway. I rushed out of the house with no makeup on, but that was not unusual if I was in a hurry. I would do it on the way or at my final destination. I told them how I never put on my make-up and that I collapsed when I got to my table at the Girl Scouts breakfast.

I told them how I was rushed to the emergency room, spent ten days in Neurological Intensive Care and a total of thirty-two days in the hospital. I told them how I literally could not talk for three-and-a-half weeks. I thanked them for their prayers because I told them that I knew Pastor had not allowed them to come to visit me, but it was for a good reason. My brain needed time to heal and did not need too much stimulation. I told them that by the grace of God, I stood before them. I received a standing ovation.

On one Sunday in January 2014, one of my church members came up to me after service and told me how touched she was by my testimony. She told me that she hoped I didn't mind, but she had shared it with someone she knew who had recently suffered a stroke and that my testimony had helped this person. I assured her that I did not mind, and that's why I had shared it. She would not be the last person to say similar words to me.

I would later tell my story in front of a crowd of attendees at a fundraiser for Aurora St. Luke's Medical Center. The event raised money for the expansion of the neurology department there to what's now called the Aurora Neuroscience Innovation Institute. It opened in early 2015. I also did television interviews with my rehabilitation specialist on one local Milwaukee TV station and by myself on my old station later that year.

Every time I share my story with women, especially what doctors believe caused my stroke—birth control pills over the age of forty—half the women seem to know of this risk while the other half were like me in the beginning, unaware that this is an issue. For example, Beverly said her doctor took her off birth control pills when she was 35. When she asked why, he told her that she was too young to have a stroke.

By November 22, 2014, a visit with my neurosurgeon ended with the news that I had made a full recovery. In early 2015, I had one last appointment at the Aurora Neuroscience Innovation Institute. I was told at that time that there was a 0.1% chance that I would have another stroke. I was removed from all prescribed medications by then, and I only had to take a baby aspirin daily.

Those who remember when my words suddenly stopped in 2013 forget that I had a stroke. Those who meet me for the first time are always shocked that I had such an experience. I literally had to find my voice again, and I am using it now to give God *all* the glory.

A Final Note

Dear Reader,

Despite my swift recovery, I think about my stroke every day. When I wake up every morning, I'm thanking God because I know how one brief moment can change the direction of one's life forever, so I am grateful.

As I get older, I often wonder if some of my memory losses are because of the natural aging process, or are they related to my stroke experience. These thoughts confronted me head-on during my first few months back at work.

I was anxious to get back to work. I started back in January 2014, but my doctor had advised that I could only work part-time. He approved me for four hours a day for the first two weeks, and six hours a day for the next two weeks, which meant I did not reach full-time until February. He was right to limit my hours. I was so exhausted during my first week back after just four hours of work that I went home and took a nap every day.

Fast forward to my days at the office in March. Surely, I was back on all cylinders. I hadn't really thought much about it until one progress meeting with my boss. For these meetings, I would always have an agenda to make sure I discussed everything I needed to share. At one point, she asked me about a task she wanted me to do, which had not been handled.

"Oh, yes. I still need to do that," I responded.

"Are you still having residual issues from your stroke?" she asked.

I was mortified. Her question stopped me cold. My mind was racing, running through a multitude of thoughts and doubts. *Do I forget things? Am I still suffering from stroke symptoms? Why have I not gotten that done? Am I still sick? I thought I was back to normal again.*

I just apologized and vowed that I would get the task done right away. The incident made me start paying closer attention to what I was doing. It made me re-think my things-to-do-lists, making sure I had completed my projects and had a satisfactory answer if I had not. I also finally realized there was a reason people who would see me for the first time after learning about my stroke would always ask about how I was feeling with a sobering tone and a grim look on their faces. Hoping people would not think I was incapable of my work, I would put on a positive face but secretly wonder, *Am I different? Am I capable?*

This seemed like a familiar pattern; the one Tracey talked to me about. The black-woman syndrome of saying, "I've got this," when maybe I didn't. I had always tried to focus on the positive, even before I attributed the positive to God. I would push negativity to the side and keep moving.

I had a conversation with my mother once and learned that she had done the same thing in her life with negative thoughts. I have learned that sometimes that's not always good. Sometimes it protects us, but often it prevents us from having real conversations about the things that are bothering us. That's probably why I never had a real conversation about sex with my mother. When I was a teenager, she had asked me to come to her when I felt like I wanted to have sex so we could get me on birth control. When I thought I was in love, I did just that. She asked *why* I needed birth control, a question I did not expect. Embarrassed, I made up an excuse and told her my friends said it helped mitigate cramps. *Really, Vivian?*

Fortunately, I have grown past that. Today, I am who I am, and I know whose I am. I try my best to be kind because people are dealing with so much strife in the world that you never know when your kind word or gesture may be the only one they've had that day. And I strive to be honest and not only live my truth but speak my truth. You can never really know when the words will suddenly stop.

Acknowledgments

So many people helped me complete this book. If I forget someone, please charge it to my stroke-ridden head and not my heart.

First, I thank God for sparing my life on October 25, 2013. He has been with me all the way and continues to be with me. In fact, He is the one who made sure that my life crossed paths with everyone else I plan to acknowledge on this page.

I thank all of the medical professionals who helped me—from the paramedics to the emergency room personnel at Aurora Sinai Medical Center, to the caregivers at the Aurora St. Luke's Neurological Intensive Care Unit, to the doctors, nurses and therapists on 2 North at St. Luke's, and finally, the therapists who helped me after my hospital stay.

I have to thank my posse again: my mother, Marilyn King; my sorority sisters, June Perry-Stevens, Joan Prince, Beverly Cooley, Jessica Murphy, Grant McLean, and Nuntiata Buck; my TV Sisterhood, Susan Kim, Katrina Cravy, Kim Buchanan-Rietbrock; and my friend, Tracey Golden.

Thank you to my Pastor and First Lady, John Wesley McVicker, Sr. and Marilynn McVicker, for your prayers and getting Christ the King Baptist Church to pray for me.

Thank you to the rest of my friends who granted me interviews for this book: Sadhna Lindvall, Genyne Edwards, Deidra Edwards, Nayo Parret, Kimberly Montgomery, Michelle Greene, Crystal McNeal, Nayo Parret, Julietta Henry, Raymond Downs and James Lynch.

My soror and fellow stroke survivor, Dana London, came up with the title I used for this book. We co-authored an article for a Delta Sigma Theta newsletter, detailing our stroke experiences, and "When the Words Suddenly Stopped" rolled off her tongue so easily. I added the sub-title, but her stroke of genius gave life to my book, and she so graciously agreed to share her idea.

Thanks to my beta readers, who took time out of their busy schedules to read my first draft and make suggestions: Crystal McNeal, Teresa Coffer, Margaret Holloway, Gina Jones and two of my posse mentioned before, Beverly Cooley, and Jessica Murphy. I hope I captured all of your thoughts and made this into a better story that will serve as inspiration for those who read it.

A huge thank you to my dear friend, Hosea Sanders. You were not able to be by my side during my ordeal as you wished, but your foreword shows just how much you are always there for and with me.

Finally, thanks to my editors, Jane VanVooren Rogers and Gailyc Braunstein, who made sure every word in this book made sense. Sharron Jewell and Gwen Mosley finished the review of this book with stellar proofreading. You all are the best.

About the Author

Vivian King is a dynamic communications leader with an extensive career in broadcast journalism, public relations, and community relations. She provides personalized consulting to individuals looking to find their voice through the media and connecting with community through workshops and forums. A native of St. Louis, Vivian received her journalism degree from the University of Missouri-Columbia. Connect with her at VivianLKing.com.

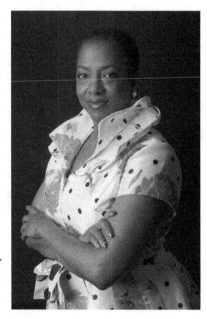

Resources

The following resources may be of assistance for researching or overcoming a stroke:

Mayo Clinic
https://www.mayoclinic.org

FAST Stroke Guide, By Dr. Akram Shhadeh
https://www.amazon.com/
FAST-Stroke-Guide-Akram-Shhadeh/dp/0578500833

Aurora Neuroscience Innovation Institute
2801 W. Kinnickinnic River Parkway, #680
Milwaukee, WI 53212
(414) 385-1922
https://www.aurorahealthcare.org/services/neuroscience

American Heart & Stroke Association
http://honor.americanheart.org/site/
PageServer?pagename=funraiser13_aboutus

Centers for Disease Control
https://www.cdc.gov

Clot Care
http://www.clotcare.com

CaringBridge
https://www.caringbridge.org

Tracey Golden, MS, LPC
Expansion Consulting
207 E. Buffalo, Suite 517
Milwaukee, WI 53202
(414) 292-9162
https://www.psychologytoday.com/us/therapists/
tracey-golden-milwaukee-wi/313896

Book Club Questions

1. What do you think was the author's motivation for this book?

2. Did the topic interest you, even if you were previously unfamiliar with it?

3. Who was your favorite character in the book?

4. Who was your least-favorite character in the book?

5. Was there a favorite story that captured your attention? If so, which one and why?

6. The "What I've Learned" Chapter mentions the three Ps. Do you have a posse? Would they be there for you in the case of an illness?

7. Are you persistent with your health? How do you advocate for yourself and your loved ones?

8. How important is prayer and your faith when handling difficult issues? How does faith play a role in your life?

9. Discuss how your mental health may impact your physical wellness.

10. Will you apply anything you learned or create a new habit because of this book?

11. How did the author find her voice?

CPSIA information can be obtained
at www.ICGtesting.com
Printed in the USA
LVHW080035250720
661378LV00017BA/1658